Finally, a smart, readable book that addresses the nutrition, exercise, and lifestyle needs of women over 50. Well-organized and easy to follow, this book is a winner. Highly recommended!

> Jonny Bowden, PhD, CNS, aka "The Nutrition Myth Buster," author of *Living Low Carb, The Great Cholesterol Myth,* and *Smart Fat: Eat More Fat. Lose More Weight. Get Healthy Now.*

In her new book, *You Still Got It, Girl! The After 50 Fitness Formula for Women,* Debra Atkinson provides a much-needed solution. Integrating the latest research from a number of disparate fields, including endocrinology, sports medicine, weight loss, nutrition, and gerontology, she outlines a novel approach to weight loss and long-term health for the over-50 crowd. An approach that's practical, do-able, and sustainable for both the exercise beginner and the fitness aficionado.

> Tamara Grand, PhD, CPT, online group and individual fitness coach at Fitknitchick.com

This book puts a significant amount of important information in a concise package, enabling the reader to discover lifestyle patterns that lead to longer and more energetic lives. The contents will be eye-opening, helping readers to dramatically and successfully change their approach to nutrition, exercise, and aging.

> Charlie Hoolihan, IDEA presenter, Pelican Athletic Club personal training director

You Still Got It, Girl! The After 50 Fitness Formula for Women is an insightful review of the reality that women face with their health, eating habits, hormones, and lifestyle. Debra presents an honest picture of how poor choices and unhealthy lifestyle practices can sabotage health and wellness. This information is followed by practical solutions and insights on how any woman can take control and enjoy what should be the best years of her life.

> Maureen Hagan, BScPT, BA PE, award-winning fitness instructor and program director

YOU STILL GOT IT, GIRL!

The After 50 Fitness Formula for Women

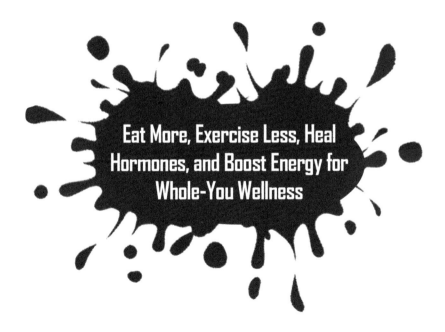

Eat More, Exercise Less, Heal Hormones, and Boost Energy for Whole-You Wellness

Debra Atkinson, MS, CSCS

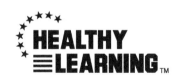

HEALTHY
LEARNING™

ISBN: 978-1-60679-346-6
Library of Congress Control Number: 2015956622
Book layout: Cheery Sugabo

Healthy Learning
P.O. Box 1828
Monterey, CA 93942
www.healthylearning.com

Dedication

To my beautiful mother

Acknowledgments

This book happened, in part, thanks to my midlife crisis. I'm thankful for the many major life changes that happened at once that forced me out of my comfortable, yet stagnant, security, and woke me up to possibilities and my dreams.

I thank my son, Dustin, for telling me to jump when I needed to hear it and for being the reason everything matters. Not surprisingly, my heart is still in the Midwest. Thanks to my family who all came running when I needed them and to my 89-year-young mom, who's still pretty hot without the flash. Thanks to TD for catching me at the finish and inspiring me every day to get there.

In the two years while I was focusing on the contents of this book, before I knew it was a book, so many women have openly shared their baffling challenges climbing hormonal mountains. My primary research came from women just like you, dear reader. The questions you asked and the frustrations you expressed led me to begin group coaching and create content to help you solve problems for which there were few answers. You deserve a second 50 that rocks.

Thank you to Dr. Jim, Kristi, and the rest of their team at Healthy Learning. They gave my thoughts and words legs. Thank you for clarifying what it was I really wanted to say and for the patience and grace with which you used your red pen.

I am grateful for a 30-year career in the Midwest, as well as the last two years in this utopia called Boulder, CO. Without one, I would not have seen the possibilities in the other. I'll leave you to guess which is which.

Thank you to Erin, Melissa, and the team they've created at Rallysport, who have given me a glance at what's possible when you find excellent people and they want to do excellent work. You can get out of the way and let it happen. Landing here gave me the room to research and write without losing touch with the working world. Watching from the outside, instead of in the storm, has given me new perspective and appreciation of unique talents.

I want to thank the clubs where I've worked in the Midwest and trainers that I've consulted with around the country. Without their additional input, I'd have developed this book with a singular vantage point. As you serve both men and women in their second 50, you're changing lives and creating legacies beyond your own. The better we serve them, the richer the world will be from their gifts.

Foreword

Being fit and 50 is not mutually exclusive. It better not be. With 75 million baby boomers, the majority of whom are women, currently journeying through their next 50 years, being mentally and physically fit is critical for successful longevity. Sister Genevieve Kunkle, a media star among the great centenarians, was once asked what was the secret to her longevity. Her answer was short and sweet. "I have but two good traits. I'm alert, and I'm vertical." Being cognitively sharp is essential for high-quality living. But equally as important is having the strength, flexibility, and balance to assume the vertical, followed by the endurance to walk to the staircase and then climb it without having to speed dial 911.

And so it goes for any woman after age 50. The reality is that you have to work a bit harder and stay consistent with simple strategies that help you to achieve and maintain a mind and body that can carry you through the challenges of the second half of your life. Here's the good news. No matter how many years you've not attended to your body's health and fitness, that same marvelous body is quite forgiving. It may not bounce back as fast as when you were twenty or thirty, but it can indeed significantly improve.

Furthermore, there's science behind this. My colleague and fellow American College of Sports Medicine scientist, Dr. Ulrik Wisloff, created a terrific online tool, the Fitness Age Test, to help monitor your progress as you begin to practice a more active lifestyle. Sitting on the board of the National Senior Games, I teamed with Ulrik to apply the test to the 11,000 athletes, all of whom are at least 50, and who qualified to compete at the 2015 Games. Lo and behold, while the average age of the men and women was 68, their fitness age was 43, or a whopping 25 years younger. As a competing Senior Olympic triathlete, I completed the test in five minutes and discovered that I, too, was a quarter century younger. Now, there's a nice payoff most individuals were not anticipating. The point is that athletes push the envelope and help us to see the outer limits and boundaries to the rewards for our fitness efforts. No one has to become a competitive athlete to reap great benefits for showing up and getting fit. Take the test, and if the result is not so great right now, then there's your incentive to get rocking on your *After 50 Fitness Formula*. It's never ever too late to get started. Soon you'll be singing, "50 is the new 40…!"

Debra Atkinson, fitness expert and champion of female boomer fitness, has created a comprehensive, easy-to-follow blueprint for women to get the *what, why,* and *how* of becoming fit after the age of 50. She'll take you on a journey through how the 50-plus woman can assess her current mental, nutritional, and physical fitness, and then how she can apply simple habits that make a world of difference. The 50-plus years are, to say the very least, a challenging roller coaster, taking women through steep hormonal peaks and valleys, mind-boggling social stresses, and body-morphing physical transformations. Instead of becoming overwhelmed by decreasing energy, an ever-widening girth, and body parts that seem to be heading south, take heart that Debra's got your back, literally. She'll support and coach you as you take your first tenuous, courageous steps toward new and healthier lifestyle choices.

Why are you, a woman who is 50-plus, doing this at all? Research has shown that the one thing women prize more than anything else as they age is their *independence*. We're fine with caregiving anyone who comes within a hundred-mile radius. But, when it comes caring for ourselves, we want to remain mentally and physically strong enough not to have people fuss over us. We pride ourselves on how well we can get out of that chair by ourselves, run after kids and grandkids, and haul the grocery bags out of our cars. If independence is such a powerful motivator, then women need to embrace and practice the lifestyle habits that will help them stay strong. How strong? Well, fit enough to save their own life if they fall and no one is available to help. After the age of 50, fitness is no longer just about looking and feeling good. It's about survival. It's also about avoiding frailty and eliminating or minimizing disability. Achieving mental and physical fitness will help you reach these goals.

Debra Atkinson is on a mission to help women who are over 50 feel hope that they can truly make simple, but significant, changes to undertake that fresh start and not only get back in the game, but win it—for life.

> Pamela M. Peeke, MD, MPH, FACP, FACSM
> Pew Foundation Scholar in Nutrition and Metabolism
> Assistant Professor of Medicine, University of Maryland
> *New York Times* bestselling author *of Fight Fat After Forty, Body-for-LIFE for Women, and The Hunger Fix: The Three-Stage Detox and Recovery Plan for Overeating and Food Addiction*

Contents

Preface

Who moved the fat? If you had time to read the overwhelming amount of conflicting advice concerning what to do to achieve a desirable level of health you're bombarded with daily, you wouldn't have time to exercise once you were done! Whether you've been exercising and eating right for years, but suddenly can't reach the intensity you used to, or can't drop those mounting pounds where your waist used to be, I've got you covered.

There is a magic secret. It's that we were wrong. We learned wrong. What we did once doesn't work and will never work again. The good news is in the last 10 years, we've learned more than in the last 50 about diet, nutrition, and five other forces that either work for or against us. In this book, you're going to learn how to have your real life, your wine, and your weight loss too.

There are many doctors, trainers, nutritionists, and books shouting their message at you. While you're running from one to the next to get pieces, you're not able to put the puzzle together. This book is your personal GPS. All the pieces are here. You'll learn where you're cruising and where you've taken an unintended wrong turn.

You'll start your journey in Chapter 1 with a checklist to target your best first step. There is one thing that, if you focus on it first, will make your ride smoother, in the right direction. You may love hearing that less sweating over exercise and eating more food than you ever thought possible is a major part of this plan. You may need to hear that rest and a massage are keys to weight loss. Whatever your experience, this book offers you a fresh start to new strategies that get you back in the game of high energy.

Introduction

If you're tired of the weight-loss, weight-gain roller coaster, overwhelmed with diet and exercise advice, and you want to avoid menopause weight gain or find a solution to low energy, high stress, stubborn pounds, and implement a smarter *complete* action plan that works and lasts, you're holding that action plan in your hands right now. How many of these problems can you identify with?

- "It doesn't matter if I eat 'good' or 'bad,' nothing seems to change."
- "I'm putting weight on in places I never had problems before."
- "I know I need to exercise, I just don't know what to do … and I don't want to get hurt."
- "Every trainer or nutritionist I see gives me different advice—whom do I believe?"
- "When I couldn't lose weight, my trainer said, 'Well, you're getting old.'"
- "I'm willing to do it, if I know what it is!"

This book will be different in two ways. First, the book brings together seven essential areas that science knows can no longer be addressed in isolation. Wonderful resource books exist for weight training, cardio, diet, sleep, stress, and hormones. Yet, none of the existing titles help you understand the integration of these pieces so you can create a whole-person fitness plan.

Second, the book will be unique from other diet or exercise books in the way it is written and formatted. It features easy-to-read type, short paragraphs and quick-read lists and sidebars so you can absorb the information quickly.

Each chapter features a different contributing expert, or case studies and success stories. You don't have to read this book front to back. You can take the assessment at the beginning of the book and then jump to the chapter you need most. Dump your thoughts of January resolutions when you've tried and failed to change everything at once. There is one thing that will have the greatest impact on your success. That's where you should begin.

The book is written in a conversational style with insightful anecdotes, checklists, and self-assessment forms. Don't let the amount of research cited scare you. The text is designed to be a blend of science and boomer-to-boomer, over-the-fence conversation. Imagine you and I having a glass of wine or cup of tea while you read. We're going to talk about cortisol as if she's not even in the room. She's not your diva.

Research on aging and every topic included in this book is exploding. My inbox is groaning. We've learned more in the last five years than in the last 30. Researchers and fitness professionals are aging too. We want answers as much as you do.

Logic will have you nodding in agreement to new information. Habit-gravity will have you pushing the same speed and incline on the treadmill as yesterday. This book provides interactive components to help you change your actions to change your results. What a waste if you only read this book and don't know what to do. I've written this book as if you are my coaching client, and we're about change.

That being said, you're an expert. I am going to encourage you to start listening to your body again. Women, in particular, have accepted symptoms and signs something is wrong as normal. The book focuses on reaching solutions naturally by defining "right" in each area. When in doubt, I encourage you to visit your local hormonitarian. Assess: don't guess. The problem with some of the things we want to test is nothing will show until you've got 90 percent damage. Trust your gut. No pun intended.

There's a Steve Jobs quote that makes regular rounds on social media. *When you look closely, most overnight successes were years in the making.* Reality is, the fatologue of belly bulge, bat wings, and kankles you're gathering didn't arrive by FedEx. It too was years in the making. What we learned and became our habits in the last 30 or more years doesn't work anymore. It never did. We were just too young and too busy to notice or to do anything about it. We just bought a bigger sweater, and more elastic waistbands, and then carpooled and climbed the ladder onward.

Chances are, if you're reading this, you're not just frustrated with being overweight or having a few extra pounds. You suffer from infobesity. This book will help you spot seductive cover headlines that blindside you when you're vulnerable and help show you what really works.

Grammar is not always followed, on purpose. You'll find a vocabulary unique to fatpedia for females. This approach is intended to be informal and more useful than proper. I hope that if you're a stickler for grammar, you'll forgive me.

Someone suggested to me that I write this book like I'm talking to a friend. I did. I don't let her off the hook too often. I'm kind of a pain like that. If she's crazy-making with excuses or sabotaging herself, it's bad enough if she believes it. I don't get in there with her. You too are going to get the science and the support, along with unbiased truth and tough love. If you're ready to put yourself first and put old ideas aside, you can feel better in your second 50 than you've ever felt in your life.

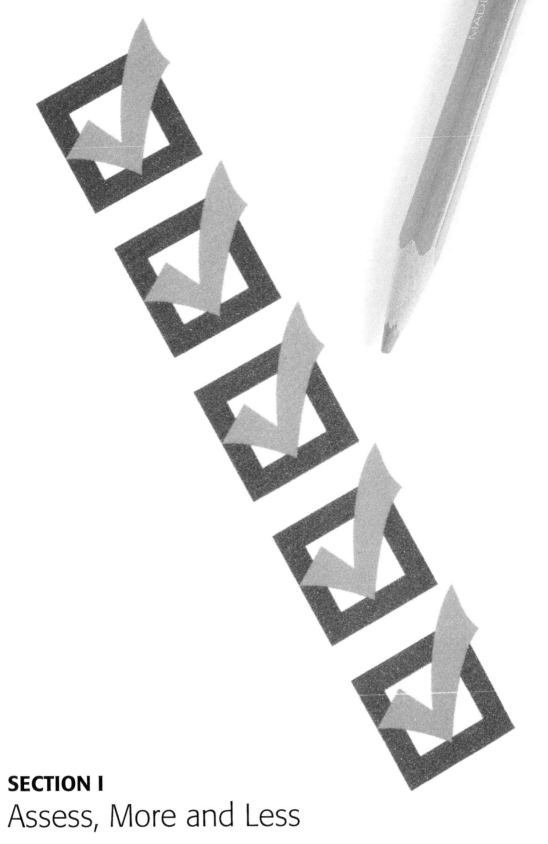

SECTION I
Assess, More and Less

The body doesn't lie.

—Martha Graham

CHAPTER 1 ————————————————————
Assess, Don't Guess

What a waste to go through a book full of fitness advice and wonder what really to do with it. The *After 50 Fitness Formula* checklist will assess your habits in each essential part of this look-good, feel-great, and reach-your-best weight plan. You'll identify what you need most. It might be action, rest, or more information through testing. When you chart your assessment scores, you'll have a clear image of where to start. While you may not yet have the answers, you will have the right questions. You can come back to this chart regularly to fill in your progress. You'll find worksheets and recording forms in the appendix to supplement each chapter. You don't have to read this book front to back. If one area calls you like a siren, head either to that chapter first or to the resources and ask questions.

Okay, grab a pencil and assess!

THE *AFTER 50 FITNESS FORMULA* CHECKLIST

A. Seven Steps: The Basics

❑ Exercise: Physical activity is consistently a part of my life.
❑ Nutrition: Eighty percent or more of the time, I choose high nutrient-dense foods.
❑ Sleep: I sleep well and wake rested daily.
❑ Stress: If I have high levels of stress, they don't negatively affect me.
❑ Hormones: I am aware of the signs and symptoms of imbalance.
❑ Rest and recovery: I plan my rest carefully, so that I have an optimal level of energy.
❑ "Wholistic" integration: I consciously adjust all six of the aforementioned areas daily.

_____ Number of boxes checked (seven maximum)

B. Exercise: Level I

❑ Cardiovascular: I do three or more cardio sessions weekly.

❑ Resistance: I do two or three strength sessions for the major muscle groups of the body weekly.

❑ Core: I perform core exercises most days of the week.

❑ Mobility: I stretch most days of the week.

_____ Number of boxes checked (four maximum)

C. Smarter Ex Rx After 50

❑ I wait at least an hour after rising before exercising.

❑ I adjust my exercise plans if I've not slept well or am sleep deprived.

❑ I always perform a warm-up that eases me into the main exercise routine I will be doing.

❑ I always stretch and perform a cool-down following my exercise session.

❑ I take at least one (or two) full day(s) off of exercising a week.

❑ I exercise according to a plan and adjust my plan, based on my energy, sleep, or stress levels, as well as my heart rate or feelings of exertion level.

❑ I regularly try new things that get me moving in different ways.

_____ Number of boxes checked (seven maximum)

D. Cardiovascular and Resistance Exercise

❑ I plan to engage in three to five cardio sessions a week.

❑ One of my cardio sessions includes intervals of high and low intensities.

❑ One of my cardio sessions is longer and slow.

❑ One of my cardio sessions is a brief moderate-to-hard challenging session (tempo).

❑ On days I don't "exercise," I get plenty of lifestyle activity.

❑ I strength train at least twice a week with a plan based on my goals and needs.

❑ I fatigue at 10 or fewer repetitions at least one day of the week, using heavy weights.

❑ I perform functional resistance exercises that vary the plane of movement and mimic activities of living at least once a week.

❑ I perform quick movements that challenge my agility, balance, and reaction motor abilities at least once a week.

_____ Number of boxes checked (nine maximum)

E. Core: The Better and Safer Flat-belly Exercises

❏ I perform core (back and ab) exercises most days of the week.

❏ I focus primarily on stabilization exercises.

❏ I also include rotation, back-extension, and lateral-flexion exercises in my routine, as well as limit the number of forward-flexion exercises I perform.

❏ I avoid crunches and sit-ups.

_____ Number of boxes checked (four maximum)

F. Mobility: The New Flexibility

❏ I either stretch, practice yoga, or do Pilates most days of the week.

❏ I focus on my hips, upper and lower back, chest, and shoulders each time I stretch.

❏ I hold stretches or poses for 15 to 30 seconds minimum.

❏ I perform static stretches, primarily after I am warmed up or after my exercise session.

_____ Number of boxes checked (four maximum)

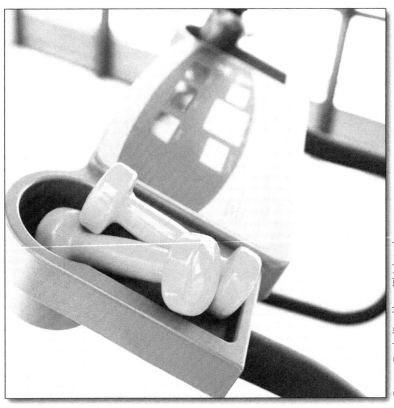

George Doyle/Stockbyte/Thinkstock

G. Medicine Cabinet in the Kitchen

❏ I eat three meals that include 25 to 30 grams of protein each day.

❏ I eat meals and snacks (if any) that combine carbs, fat, and protein.

❏ I limit my consumption of food, drinks, and snacks that are high in simple sugars.

❏ I limit my consumption of processed food, (i.e., that have been altered in some way from their natural state).

❏ I drink 6 to 10 glasses of water a day, based on my personal need.

❏ I rarely exercise on an empty stomach and fuel my exercise sessions thoughtfully.

❏ I often consume easy-to-digest protein before strength training (24 grams).

❏ I consume a 1:3 or 1:4 (protein:carb) snack within 30 minutes of exercise and/or a meal of 25 to 30 grams of protein within 90 minutes following vigorous exercise.

❏ I eat healthy fats daily (Omega 3 higher than Omega 6).

❏ I limit alcoholic drinks to one per day (for women) and eliminate them entirely if appropriate.

_____ Number of boxes checked (10 maximum)

H. Dietary Mental Medicine Cabinet

❏ I focus on eating a variety of high-quality, nutrient-dense foods.

❏ I know and practice eating that reflects the fact that *fat does not make me fat.*

❏ I avoid drinking alcohol on an empty stomach or before I've made a decision about my next meal.

❏ I always eat breakfast as one of my 3 x 25 to 30 g protein meals.

❏ I focus on drinking water *between* meals and just drink to eat comfortably at meals.

❏ I leave two or more hours between my last meal and bedtime.

❏ I don't "diet" or count calories: I make calories count.

❏ I take time to plan meals and snacks I love, I look forward to, and that give me energy.

❏ I find food pleasurable and a social experience: I've made peace with it.

❏ I don't play that exercise-so-I-can-eat or exercise-to-burn-it-off game, ever.

_____ Number of boxes checked (10 maximum)

I. Sleep

❑ I love pillow talk: I love my mattress, my sheets, and my pajamas.

❑ I have ideal sleep temperatures: my body temp and my room temp.

❑ I control any potential intrusive sound that might wake me.

❑ I remove light and keep my room dark.

❑ I remove or eliminate LED and screens 90 minutes before bedtime.

❑ I have a sleep-cues routine.

❑ I get seven to nine hours of sleep at night (or know my optimal number of sleep hours and get it).

❑ I pass the wake-naturally-feel-rested test.

_____ Number of boxes checked (eight maximum)

J. Stress

❑ I know my environmental stressors and either eliminate or reduce them.

❑ I regularly socialize, vent, and enjoy friendships.

❑ I connect with family and friends at least once daily.

❑ I have a sense of purpose about what I'm doing here.

❑ I have a belly laugh every day.

❑ I surround myself with beauty in art, color, nature, or music every day.

❑ I know my emotional stressors and try to reduce my exposure to them.

❑ I choose healthy ways to relieve stress.

❑ I know my stress signs and symptoms and respond quickly with my personal 911.

_____ Number of boxes checked (nine maximum)

K. Hormone Hell-O

❑ Cortisol: I know the symptoms of cortisol imbalance.

❑ Insulin: I understand how foods trigger insulin and what happens after that occurs.

❑ Ghrelin: I know what ghrelin is and how it affects weight gain.

❑ Leptin: I know what leptin does and how it affects weight gain.

❑ Estrogen-progesterone-testosterone: I understand the necessary balance of these three sex hormones and the signs that they might not be in balance.

❑ DHEAs: I know what this factor is and how a deficiency might show up.

❑ Adrenals: I understand the signs and symptoms of adrenal fatigue.

❑ Thyroid: I know the relationship between adrenals and thyroid and the right questions to ask about lifestyle adjustment.

❑ I've discussed these hormones and assessed with my physician (if needed).

❑ I understand the role each hormone plays and how they interact with each other for weight gain, loss, or energy.

_____ Number of boxes checked (nine maximum)

L. Rest and Recovery

❑ I add my life work, physical work and play, and emotional stress levels to determine my total allostatic load.

❑ I know the difference between good tired, fatigue, and lethargy.

❑ I know what it means to fully recharge my batteries.

❑ I plan rest and recovery, rather than waiting until I *need* it.

_____ Number of boxes checked (four maximum)

M. Whole-You Approach

❑ I am working with my allostatic load and my goals in an integrated way.

❑ I live as if there's no way to isolate mind-body-spirit any more.

❑ I don't wait for the spirit to move me: motion drives emotion.

❑ I seek someone else's insight when the little b---- inside my head isn't supportive or helping me get results.

❑ I want to and am willing to *make changes* so I see and feel changes.

_____ Number of boxes checked (five maximum)

Total score _____ (90 maximum)

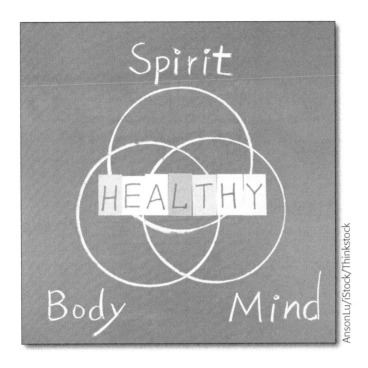

AnsonLu/iStock/Thinkstock

INSTRUCTIONS FOR THE CHECKLIST

- Respond to each statement. If the statement is true for you, check the box. If it isn't 100 percent true, leave it blank until you have done the work or made changes so it's true. Be tough with your grading. Your results depend on it!
- Summarize each section. Add the number of checked boxes for each section. Note your current total: _____. Fill in the boxes in Figure 1-1 for each corresponding section.

	A	B	C	D	E	F	G	H	I	J	K	L	M
10	█	█	█	█	█	█			█	█	█	█	█
9	█	█	█		█	█			█			█	█
8	█	█	█		█	█						█	█
7		█	█									█	█
6		█	█		█	█						█	█
5		█	█		█							█	
4													
3													
2													
1													

Figure 1-1. The *After 50 Fitness Formula* checklist scorecard

- Consider the sections where you had the lowest percentage of checks areas on which to focus. Cross out those items that don't apply to you. If, for instance, due to a condition you have or a medication you might be taking, one of the items may not be possible, then eliminate it. (Fill in that box on the grid also.)
- Keep playing until you can check all the boxes. Books, programs, coaches, videos, and friends may all be a part of your toolkit. It might take a week to fill them all in. It might take a year. Changing habits (and changing thoughts in order to do *that*) is not for wimps. Be up for the job!
- Give yourself credit as you get points from each category. Fill in the columns from the bottom up. You'll gain knowledge of each essential area in the chapters that follow. Visit http://foreverfitandfab.com for more information.
- As you go through each chapter, revisit the checklist frequently. What gets measured matters. The more you turn your focus to learning why what you're doing isn't working, or reinforce what is, the closer you'll be to the results you want.

All of the elements on the checklist affect you and your ability to find your optimal *After 50 Fitness Formula*. Figure 1-2 shows what you already know. Sleep affects you. Nutrition affects you. Until now, you may not have planned rest and recovery until the need hit you hard, but you knew you needed it. How can you change your diet to affect your sleep? How can you change your exercise to positively affect your hormones?

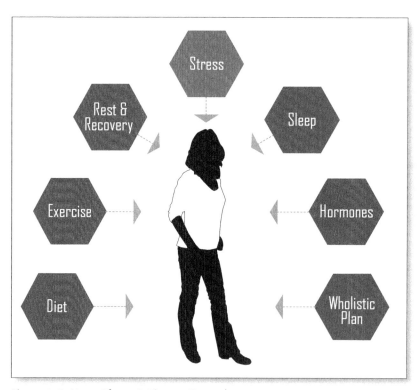

Figure 1-2. Your *After 50 Fitness Formula* components

Which of those changes should you focus on first? That's what you're going to find out. Now that you're aware of the importance of these individual parts, you need to look at their integration. Figure 1-3 illustrates that each of the elements of your *After 50 Fitness Formula* affects the others. You're about to learn how to bring them together optimally for your personal fitness formula.

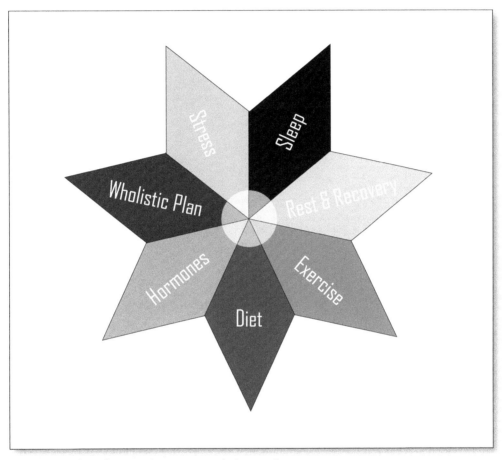

Figure 1-3. The *After 50 Fitness Formula* integration

Not everything that can be counted counts.

—Albert Einstein

CHAPTER 2 —————————————————————————

Stop Counting Calories and Make Calories Count

This book is not your mother's diet book. The use of the word diet from this point on is not the four-letter word version that has an exit ramp. This approach is just a reaffirmation of the lifetime practice required for consuming fuel with pleasure. The foods you love have to be included.

You may be a vegetarian. You may be a meat-lover. You may choose not to eat gluten or not tolerate dairy. No one-size-fits-all diet exists. You have a unique biochemistry like no one else. This chapter aims to give you a basis for making choices and decisions. Think about whether omitting a complete food group is a good idea. This chapter will show you how foods affect you in a systematic way.

You're subject to articles, blogs, books, and documentaries that tell you meat is bad, meat is good; vegetables are good, nightshade vegetables are bad; dairy is good for bones, dairy doesn't matter for bones, ad nauseam, It's exhausting! This chapter provides you with research and the professional opinion of nutrition and medical experts so you can make more informed decisions about what you put in your mouth.

Most women who reach 50 have probably done the following. You go on a diet, reduce your caloric intake for weeks, exercise like a crazy boot-camp kamikaze six days a week, lose weight, end your participation in diet and boot camp, and then hope things work out for you. Data show, short-term diets have a failure rate of 95 percent. You may have read that most dieters fail. Wrong. It's not your fault.

There is actually evidence to suggest that the chemical reactions in your body set you up to fail. It isn't that you weren't disciplined enough or were too lazy. Physiological responses to reducing weight make you gain weight. Your body turns up the volume on hunger. It decreases the amount of energy you expend. Stress responses in your body make you store more fat. On a typical jump-on-the-treadmill, slash-calories approach, you're doomed.

Biologically, your calorie intake and calorie expenditure are coupled. Your super-smart system naturally tries to decrease energy expenditure when you decrease calories. It gives you more cravings and hunger pangs. Scientists call this driving compensatory overcompensation. You might call it wanting dessert first, second, and third course, no matter how many salads you have waiting in the refrigerator.

There are hundreds of thousands of dieting resources. They include a lot of what to avoid. In fact, it's what diets are. The five-foods-you-should-never-eat headline is marketing persuasion at its best. You can't help yourself when you click on it.

Even the nutrition content you'll find recommended in this book doesn't completely dodge what to avoid. The positive spin here is to focus on what you can do. When you think about the things you can't have, they're all you want. You start a diet focused on deprivation. How is that motivating? There are 5000 other foods and food combinations that you *can* have. Why not look there? If you take the diet highway, there is always going to be an exit ramp. Start thinking lifestyle change. This mindset is your new forever mindset.

Let's get clear. Diets work. Short-term. If you're over 50 though, even short-term diet success is harder to make happen. If you've been down that road too many times, you've been telling your body to burn fewer calories. It listened. You're left with a body that can't burn even what it once could. What follows is a typical email from a frustrated client. Does it resonate with you?

> *I'm 58, and I lost 15 pounds when I was 50. Even then, I was still about 15 pounds overweight. I just couldn't lose any more. I now have this belly fat that seems to be permanent. I can't seem to lose weight unless I go below 1200 calories. I'd like to exercise, but I have no energy. Is there an optimal level of protein, carbs, and fat for a woman in her 50s?*

This scenario is a perfect example of emails and letters that women write every day. With the limited amount of aforementioned information, it's impossible to give an adequate response. Yet, the low-calorie diet, coupled with no mention of protein and strength training to offset muscle losses, suggests that the weight the individual lost was largely lean muscle. When that happens, metabolism slows. The body burns fewer and fewer calories. Having a lack of energy to exercise would be normal. The body has decided low-energy expenditure is necessary. A return to a "normal" pattern of eating is going to result in additional weight gain—primarily of fat.

This story can still have a happy ending, however. If you're wondering, *"Can I lose the weight I've gained since menopause?"* the answer is, *"Can you lose the thoughts you gained about weight loss before menopause?"* If you can, you can absolutely have more energy and fewer inches in your future.

Everything you do has either a positive or negative impact on your metabolism. If you spent time looking for the secret, the easy solution, the fast fix, you missed the easy answer right before your eyes. Find good-for-you food that tastes good, satisfies, and balances your hormones.

Consider everything that you put into your mouth either medicine or poison. How would that change things? Do you ever consider that a little arsenic would be appropriate? Just a little sliver?

If you have ever dieted, lost weight, and then returned to the normal diet pattern that got you to the place where you needed to lose weight in the first place, you got fatter in that cycle. Dieting causes a loss of both muscle and fat, even in the best of conditions. You can lose as much as 50 percent muscle. When you gain back weight after a diet, as 66 percent of dieters do, you gain back nearly 100 percent fat. If you're diligent with strength training and adequate protein, you can recoup your muscle losses. Few women do that with focus, while they are either driving the mini-van, leaping through aerobics, or sitting in the boardroom.

The number one predictor of weight gain is a history of dieting. Weight regain after a diet often surpasses the loss. The reason is complicated and simple—all at the same time. Your body is comfortable at "home." Set point is the term you've heard in the past.

Your body burns a certain number of calories to keep you going. If you feed it fewer calories, the message you're sending is "burn fewer calories." So, it does. Then, you go back to eating a normal amount of calories and the occasional splurge. If you lost weight, you now have less muscle mass. Your body can get by on fewer calories. So, it simply stores the excess you give it as fat. It's your rainy-day fund. For you, now, it potentially feels like hurricane season. It came on slowly, but together with hormones, stressors, and just a little more time to think about life and health, you want it off yesterday.

The big message at this point is if you want long-term health and energy, you won't diet. You will change your diet. Stop using diet as a four-letter word. Your chance of being your slim self (it might never be size two or four or even six; get over it), having energy, and glowing, is rooted in your nutrition. If you're an exercise hater, that's OK. The secret is really in the way you eat. Eat more of the right foods. Exercise is your condiment. If, on the other hand, you love to exercise, you can eat more, because you move more. You do have to be careful of overcompensating. You don't have more cake. You have a lot more kale and a little more sweet potato. The time you add extra calories is on your training days around your exercise and recovery time.

Recent books on the market by medical professionals and wellness experts use the term "diet" in the title, because it sells. By the time you're 50, your female brain is programmed to equate the word diet with skinny, slim, and slender. These new books tend to detail ways of eating, as well as nutritionally sound systems for reaching optimal health. You'll find several listed in the resources section. In order to get them in your hands, the wisdom of publishers and marketers is that the title has to be juicy and appealing. Diets sell the dream.

It's ironic how a diet starts in hope and results in failure. Don't let that eternal optimism escape you. If you've dieted and lost weight, but you've gained it back, and you're not at your ideal weight, it didn't work. Women will often say, "The only way I can lose weight is to count calories." Are you losing fat? If the calorie counting works so well, why do you have to do it again?

Focus on behavior change. Make choices, not for a 21-day challenge or a 30-day diet, but forever. That said, you do have to address first what's not working under your hood. Like spinach, one of the most nutrient-rich foods available, isn't a good choice when you have the stomach flu. The best exercise and food plan won't work until you get hormones working well. There's one exception to making dietary changes. A temporary change in the types of food you eat, without a restriction in calories, has helped many women, and it can help you.

If you're waiting for the menu suggestions and the recipes, there will be few in this book. Overall, the focus of this book is on a pattern of eating. You need to make peace with food first. Then, you can learn how to eat. Then, the Google recipe file is your friend, not the devil.

Do you have a fascination with recipes? Most women do. You probably spend a lot of time thinking, planning, preparing, eating, and guilting over food.

Women who reach out for help will often say, *"I'm ready, I'll do whatever I need to do … but not on the weekends."* If this person is you, you're looking at diet as a punishment. You're not really ready for permanent change. Until you decide eating well and right is not deprivation, but a gift of well-being and the bring-sexy-back, skin-glowing secret you're looking for, you'll start and stop. Adapting a lifestyle doesn't mean that you can't have a piece of birthday cake. It just means you'll think twice, have a smaller piece, savor it if it's worth it, and move on. You may even pass on it, and you'll have a different mindset.

If 80 percent of the time, you eat based on taste and high-nutrient density, you will experience high energy and enhanced sleep. When you color outside the lines up to 20 percent of the time, you'll enjoy it. Your sensitivity to "treats" will be unique to you. You may feel "food hangover" after a weekend away indulging, while someone else doesn't even notice. When you deviate from foods that make you feel amazing and notice the difference, it's a good sign. It reinforces how very worthwhile your right choices are.

A recent study suggests that it is normal for weight to fluctuate day to day. Monday and Tuesday weight is predictably higher, but returns to a normal weight, when subjects resume their weekday eating regimen. That's acceptable and normal. This book isn't suggesting that you splurge or have binge days. This book suggests you identify foods that make you feel great and those that don't. Dieting elicits negative emotions tied to depression. Ditch the diet mentality.

A scale can be a friend or foe. If you weigh yourself, pick a day of the week and stick to it. If you want to see your weekly low, don't weigh yourself on Monday morning. Weigh if you must, later in the week. Remember that unless that scale tells you both your body fat and weight, then it doesn't tell the whole story. As a woman over 50, you don't want to see weight go down and your body fat percentage go up. A loss of muscle mass means that over time, you'll burn fewer calories, have less tone, and sabotage your weight for the future.

Jumping on the scale can increase your cortisol level. Data finds that it can be stressful, even when you don't think so. Subsequently, this stress ends up being a part of diet failure. Cortisol doesn't help you lose weight; it helps you hold and store more fat. That's physiological, and it's happening in your body, even if you don't feel stressed about it. That's why you might persevere and push through a restrictive diet that, in the end, will make you gain more fat.

Eating is enjoyable and pleasurable. At the least, it has the potential to be. You may be someone who thinks of food as fuel and not much more. Maybe you're a foodie, with recipes, meal-planning, pinning, posting, and sharing your way to food pleasures. Either way, the next chapter has you covered. Sit-downs, make-ahead meals, and shortcuts all fit.

Do something so totally for you and selfish that it might hurt. Stop counting calories. By calorie counting, you are encouraged to eliminate flavor, pleasure, and the health benefits of higher-calorie, higher-fat foods that actually help you lose inches, weight, and fatigue.

The first law of thermodynamics is wrong. Different diets lead to different biochemical pathways. Biologically speaking, a calorie is not a calorie. In plain English, some calories tend to be more easily stored as fat, and some do not. Calorie counting doesn't predict fat loss, as much as reduced simple carbohydrate consumption does.

Certain foods can give you a metabolic advantage. Think of it as metabolic inefficiency. While you may be trying to make everything else in your life run well, you want your body to run inefficiently. You can help it *burn* more calories due to heat, instead of providing more energy that, left unused, goes to your thighs.

Getting metabolically inefficient means you can eat more calories and still lose weight. They have to be the right calories, and we're not talking celery and carrot sticks alone. Juicy salmon, crunchy nuts, and creamy avocado are several of these weight loss- inducing friends high in calories, but with a positive influence on the sexy you waiting to be introduced to the world.

Why not decide to go on the saggy-skin, fatigue-loss diet? When you choose foods with the highest nutrient density, your skin, eyes, and hair will respond. Your brain will work better. Shifting to "how much health does it have," instead of "how many calories or fat does it have," will be difficult. You won't be able to help yourself. You'll say, "I thought that had so many calories." It might. So what? Your hormones rule your weight-loss world, not your calories.

If you want to be a loser—a biggest weight, inches, or baggage loser—healthy fat is your friend. Healthy fat includes all but trans-fats. Yes, even those made-villainous saturated fats have health benefits.

There is a good chance that everything that you have been taught about losing weight is wrong. The habits and thoughts you have about diet, exercise, and weight loss, acquired in the first decades of your adult life, have been proven wrong. That doesn't make new ideas easy to adopt. You have a habit gravity that makes you revert to the same choices.

You will read the ideas and suggestions based on facts, case studies, and research in this book. You'll nod your head at the logic. Then, pulling foods out of the refrigerator or ordering off a menu, you will make choices based on your old habits. It will take time. Allow yourself the time to adapt. Short-term resets can be helpful. Yet, three days or even two weeks of change won't shake three decades easily.

A linear march right to better habits and optimal weight would be wonderful. Read that as too good to be true. Behavior change takes repeated failures. Allow them. Changing permanently is not a stair-step, but a cyclic process. On average, it takes about seven attempts to learn from what didn't work, and then move to the next level.

Habits take 66 days to make or break. You're probably going to do both. You will find habits you need to stop and new habits with which you want to replace them. Don't let anyone tell you three weeks or 21 days is enough to make change. It's a myth that started, got passed on, and perpetuated, like gossip in junior high. You need to use the information in this book to make it easy to succeed and hard to fail during those 66 days and beyond. Don't bring into your house what you don't want to eat. If you decide you want or need a treat, you can go get it. You can order a serving of it and be done with it. It doesn't need to be conveniently available in the freezer.

What do you do about other members in the family? The truth is that you're the velvet hammer. Women rule the boardroom, the bedroom, and the kitchen. You have more influence on the health and wellness choices of everyone living under your roof than anything or anyone else. If you teach your family that a menopausal woman needs a certain kind of calories and better health, but they can eat carbage and crap, you set them up for the same cycle you're going through.

Sure, someone else might need more calories, and more energy for growth or activity. Do they need low-quality calories? At the least, feed them the good stuff first. You can find ways to help all of you get healthier, think better, look better, and feel better. That's a gift, not the food police.

If you've been so concerned about weight loss that you've ignored whether you lost fat or muscle, you have your work cut out for you. Changing your mind is your first hurdle. Only then will changing your body happen. If you lose muscle, you will become fatter than before the diet.

If you eat the right foods, studies show up to 97 percent of the weight you lose can be fat. By coupling the right exercise with the right nutrition, you can both lose fat and gain lean muscle. With most popular diets, this scenario is almost unheard of.

Your job, then, is to identify what are the right foods for you. There are unique differences about how foods affect you, based on your biochemistry, your stress level, and your lifestyle habits. The *After 50 Fitness Formula* you arrive at will look different than anyone else's.

There are definitely some common themes that apply to both you and your girlfriends. In the following chapter, you'll learn how lower *glycemic-load* (not glycemic-index) foods positively influence body weight and your energy expenditure, independently of caloric intake. You can eat 1000 calories (not recommended) of fruits or 1000 calories of lean protein and non-starchy vegetables. Data indicate that you could gain fat weight on the high fruit diet, even with the low-calorie count, because of its impact on insulin and the other hormones affecting appetite and fat storage.

Sugars and refined starches, like white rice and foods with white flour, cause blood sugar to rise, and insulin levels then respond in kind. A rapid drop in blood sugar causes cravings, even if physiologically you don't need more food to function.

It's not the number of calories, but the quality of the calories that you consume that matter. Foods with empty calories have few vitamins, minerals, and fiber and are foods you want to avoid in favor of nutrient-dense calories that are high in vitamin, mineral, and fiber content per calorie.

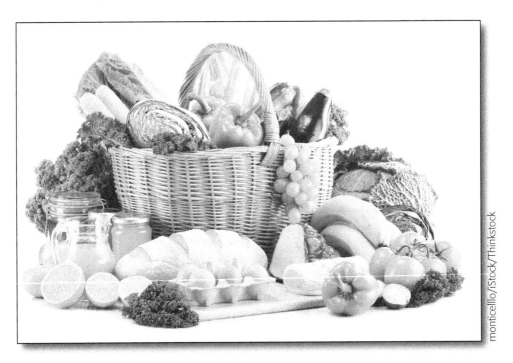

monticellio/iStock/Thinkstock

Even "healthy" foods with vitamins, minerals, and fiber—if they're concentrated sources of rapidly absorbed sugars and starches—can cause metabolic dysfunction. They can be your "crack." Fruit juice is one of these. Many "green drinks" also fit in this category.

Evidence is mounting that higher fat diets and higher calorie fattier foods produce and sustain weight loss as well as or better than calorie-restricted or higher carb diets. That's especially true if you already have metabolic abnormalities. That factor is potentially the case if you've been on that diet roller coaster of weight-on, weight-off and your metabolism is a hot mess.

You exercise telling your body to burn more calories and boost metabolism. Then, you deprive it of calories telling it to burn fewer calories and to slow its metabolism. You've put your body under a lot of stress, no doubt leading to more release of cortisol, your optimal-weight sexy-self nemesis.

Read and reread this logical thinking and science. Food is emotional. Birth, illness, graduation, weddings, death—all major events in our lives are marked with food. You can learn how to experience it all without sabotaging your health. Boomer baby, it's time to eat.

FEATURED EXPERT

Jonathan Bailor, Author of the Bestselling Book, *The Calorie Myth*

Despite the fact that virtually every lasting healthy lifestyle food-related choice (e.g., whole foods, paleo, vegetarian, low-carb, low-glycemic, Mediterranean, etc.) focuses on *what* we eat rather than *how much* we eat, the mainstream still seems to insist that if we just counted our calories more conservatively, we could end the obesity epidemic. The proven fact is that calorie-counting approaches fail 95.4 percent of the time. That's a higher failure rate than quitting smoking cold turkey.[1–4]

❑ Just Breathe Less

Blindly eating less to cure obesity is like breathing less to cure allergies. It may offer temporary "relief," but ultimately fails, because it is masking symptoms, rather than fixing causes. Will eating only 1,200 of anything cause you to lose weight? Yes. So will cutting off your leg. That doesn't mean either is a good idea. Counting calories is a euphemism for starvation. It's the definition of an eating disorder.[5] And the sooner you are able to free yourself from oppressive calorie myths, and instead enjoy eating more—but higher-quality food—the sooner you will live your best life.

❑ How to Free Yourself From Oppressive Calorie Myths

Shifting the focus from calorie quantity to food quality is easier said than done, considering the constant barrage of calorie myths we're hit with daily. To help you free yourself from disproven calorie math, the following are six of my favorite commonsense reasons calorie counting cannot be required for long-term health and fitness:

- *Nobody knew what a calorie was before the obesity epidemic.* If we need to constantly count calories to avoid obesity, then how did we have about 10 times less obesity before anyone knew what a calorie was, let alone count them?[6–8]

- *Every other species avoids obesity without counting calories.* If we need to constantly count calories to avoid obesity, how does every other animal on the planet avoid obesity even though they cannot count?

- *We don't need to count anything else we eat.* If we need to constantly count calories to avoid obesity, why don't we need to count everything else? What about vitamin C in and vitamin C out? How about zinc in and zinc out? And what about counting the other 18 minerals, 12 vitamins, nine essential amino acids, eight conditionally essential amino acids, and the two essential fatty acids?

- *No other life sustaining bodily function needs to be counted.* If we need to constantly count calories to avoid obesity, then why don't we need to "count" blood sugar to avoid diabetes? Or what about "counting" blood pressure to avoid hypertension? And how is it that when we take more water in, more water out happens unconsciously?

- *It is impossible to count calories in.* The only way to actually count calories in the real world would be to only eat food that has nutrition facts labels on them. Even in this impossible case, these labels have a 10 percent margin of error.[9] While this number may not seem like a big deal, considering that the average person eats about a million calories per year, and 10 percent of a million is 100,000 calories margin of error, which translates into 30 pounds worth of body fat, couldn't we each gain 30 pounds of fat per year even after counting every calorie we ate due to measurement error?

- *It is impossible to count calories out.* If we need to constantly count calories to avoid obesity, then how do we accurately account for the 400 to 700 calories our liver burns daily? Or what about the 200 to 400 calories we burn digesting food daily? And how do we count the 100 to 700 calories we burn per day building and repairing bodily tissue? Seventy-five percent of the calories we burn every day have nothing to do with exercise, walking, or anything measured by any expensive fitness gadget. How are we supposed to accurately and practically keep track of these?[10–12]

❑ The Flat Earth Theory of Weight Loss

Counting calories is the flat earth theory of weight loss. It's reasonable. It's intuitive. But it is wrong, once we understand modern science. The research is clear, and the common sense is undeniable. Every single society and species that ever existed that focused on foods found directly in nature—as opposed to processed low-calorie, edible products—stayed slim without counting calories. Similarly, when cultures or creatures start eating processed edible products, they start seeing increasing rates of obesity and diabetes.

Ending obesity is not about eating less or exercising more, just like ending depression is not about frowning less and smiling more. Both health and happiness are about quality, not quantity. They are about filling ourselves with so much good that we don't have room for bad. It's what we did prior to the obesity and diabetes epidemics, and it's what we'll do to end them. No math needed.

References

1. Crawford D, Jeffery RW, French SA. Can anyone successfully control their weight? Findings of a three year community-based study of men and women. *Int J Obes Relat Metab Disord*. 2000 Sep;24(9):1107-10. PubMed PMID: 11033978.
2. Summerbell CD, Cameron C, Glasziou PP. WITHDRAWN: Advice on low-fat diets for obesity. Cochrane Database Syst Rev. 2008 Jul 16;(3):CD003640. Review. PubMed PMID: 18646093.
3. Pirozzo S, Summerbell C, Cameron C, Glasziou P. Should we recommend low-fat diets for obesity? Obes Rev. 2003 May;4(2):83-90. Review. Erratum in: *Obes Rev*. 2003 Aug;4(3):185. PubMed PMID: 12760443.
4. "A word about quitting success rates." American Cancer Society: *Information and Resources for Cancer: Breast, Colon, Prostate, Lung and Other Forms*. N.p., n.d. Web. 11 Jan. 2011.
5. Diagnostic and statistical manual of mental disorders: DSM-5. 5th ed. Washington, D.C.: American Psychiatric Association, 2013. Print.
6. http://www.who.int/mediacentre/factsheets/fs311/en
7. http://www.prb.org/Articles/2002/HowManyPeopleHaveEverLivedonEarth.aspx
8. http://www.google.com/publicdata/directory
9. Urban LE, Dallal GE, Robinson LM, Ausman LM, Saltzman E, Roberts SB. The accuracy of stated energy contents of reduced-energy, commercially prepared foods. *J Am Diet Assoc*. 2010 Jan; 110(1):116-23. PubMed PMID: 20102837; PubMed Central PMCID: PMC2838242.
10. Wang Z, Heshka S, Zhang K, Boozer CN, Heymsfield SB. Resting energy expenditure: systematic organization and critique of prediction methods. *Obes Res*. 2001 May;9(5):331-6. Review. PubMed PMID: 11346676.
11. 1998: Poehlman E T; Melby C Resistance training and energy balance. *International journal of sport nutrition*. 1998;8(2):143-59.
12. Whitehead, Saffron A.; Nussey, Stephen (2001). Endocrinology: an integrated approach. Oxford: BIOS. pp. 122. ISBN 1-85996-252-1.

Jonathan Bailor is a New York Times *bestselling author and internationally recognized wellness expert, who specializes in using modern science and technology to simplify health. Bailor has collaborated with top scientists for more than 10 years to analyze and apply over 1,300 studies. His work has been endorsed by top physicians and scientists from Harvard Medical School, Johns' Hopkins, The Mayo Clinic, The Cleveland Clinic, and UCLA.*

Bailor is also the founder of SANESolution.com and serves as the CEO for the wellness technology company Yopti. He authored the New York Times *and* USA Today *bestselling book* The Calorie Myth, *hosts a popular syndicated health radio show,* The SANE Show, *and blogs on* The Huffington Post. *In addition, Bailor has registered over 25 patents, spoken at several Fortune 100 companies, as well as at the renowned TED conferences for over a decade, and served as a senior program manager at Microsoft, where he helped create Nike+ Kinect Training and XBox Fitness.*

Let food be thy medicine and medicine be thy food.

—Hippocrates

CHAPTER 3 —————————————————————
What's Fit to Eat?

The wrong foods can lead to inflammation, depression, ADD, dementia, heart disease, cancer, diabetes, and obesity. As inconvenient as your belly fat may be, it could be a sign of something worse. Yet, your start doesn't determine your end. The right foods prevent and heal.

Calories matter, but not in the simple math you grew to know. The kinds of calories you consume affect your hormones more than the number of calories. The status of your hormones regulates appetite, satiety, energy, and fat storage. Those hormones are the gatekeepers.

If you choose the type of calories you eat based on quality, you can eat up to 300 calories more a day without weight gain. In fact, a recent study showed subjects on a high-quality content diet lost more weight and gained lean muscle than subjects who ate less, but lower-quality foods.

The basic formula for choosing foods and timing them so that they optimally affect your hormones is fairly straightforward. In that regard, several general guidelines exist that apply to everyone. For example, there are your personal signs and symptoms telling you how your body is responding. Use all of the tools in your toolbox. Pay close attention to how you feel. If you've spent the last few decades paying a lot of attention to others at home and work, it's time to tune into you.

Appendix A provides worksheets for tracking your progress. Consider wiping your slate clean with one to three weeks of an elimination diet. This diet is not an effort to reduce calories and promote extreme or rapid weight loss. No, no, no. Rather, this undertaking is a brief period of time where you let your body, as well as your gut, heal and then experiment with reintroduction of foods known to be most inflammatory to determine how you respond.

The elimination diet has some side effects. You may feel withdrawal from foods to which you're practically "addicted." The stronger your reaction, the more likely that's true. There's more. You might lose inches, bloat, or pounds following this diet. You might find greater energy. Be prepared.

The following are the basics. In that regard, the rest of the chapter provides additional information.

- Protein is your lean-body best friend. Build meals around high-quality lean protein sources. If you're vegan, while this step may be harder, it is possible. Contrary to popular belief, Americans, especially older adults, do not get enough protein.
- Sugar is a big fat health and weight problem. Eliminate sugar where it's directly added and where it's hidden in "healthy" foods. Know your sugar aliases and artificial sweeteners before you simply swap one poison for another. At the present time, stevia (a sweetener extracted from the leaves of a plant) stands alone on the safe list. The After 50 Pantry Raid in Appendix A-1 details a list of items you want to avoid.
- Carbohydrates are not the enemy, if you choose carefully. The right time and type of carbohydrates improves your energy and hormone healing.
- Wine is not a food group. Resveratrol (a compound found largely in the skins of red grapes) does have health benefits, but overall, alcohol inhibits your weight loss and hormone healing. If you choose it or reintroduce it, plan carefully so you can have your wine without weight gain.
- Fat enhances fullness, satisfaction, and energy burning. Don't vilify fat, even saturated fat. Friend your fats.
- Fiber, together with protein, will help you decrease cravings. Fiber is your toxins' personal escort out of your body, fast, before they do more harm.
- Doctors (MD, PhD, NDs) and nutritionists today recommend supplements for almost everyone. Your signs, symptoms, and lifestyle can help you determine which ones you might need. When in doubt, test, don't guess. You'll find a list of supplement solutions in Appendix B-7.

If you control diet quality, quantity takes care of itself. How do you react to such a statement? If you struggle with emotional eating, you know that this statement isn't as simple as those 10 words imply. Don't expect an overnight change in ideas that took decades to establish. If you've been substituting rich foods for a rich life, you need to deal with that. Connect your emotions and your eating by journaling.

Calorie restriction is not the answer. Most recent studies reinforce this point, as well as the fact that if you're overweight or obese, it's not habit or sloth, laziness, or anything of the like. Repeat: you are not to blame. It's a physiological response that occurs with calorie cutting that causes the cascade of hormones that make you hit the weight-loss brick wall.

All the psychological food and exercise coaching in the world won't overcome a physiological problem. Your new process has to be different than that of your past in order for better results to occur. You are to blame if you diet like it's 1999 and want to be sexy in your 50s, 60s, and 70s today. So what's a hungry after 50 chic to eat?

SETTING THE STAGE: ALKALINE VS. ACIDIC FOODS

How's your pH? Your pH refers to the level of acidity or alkalinity in your body. The best state for you is slightly more alkaline than neutral. You can check your pH with litmus paper strips that test saliva or urine. Get them at vitamin stores or pharmacies. Use the five-day pH tracking form in Appendix A-9. If your body is working under too much stress in an acidic state, it can't do it's job very well.

A quick look—though nothing is that simple—at what foods cause more acidity will tell you that the average American has a highly acidic diet. Even the recommendations you're going to get soon will include acid-forming foods. A partial list of acid-forming foods includes animal protein, dairy, most beans, sugar, and sweet potatoes. Alkali-forming foods include most vegetables, azuki and lima beans, Brazil nuts, buckwheat, and barley.

You can't avoid acid-forming foods completely. You need those lean proteins. Sweet potatoes provide good carbs. Don't label foods "bad" or good. They just require an awareness of what else you're doing. The best prescription for improving your pH is to increase your intake of vegetables. A lot. Another option is to start your day with lemon water. Though lemon is an acidic food, it has an alkalizing effect on your body. With regard to enhancing your level of Ph, the following steps could be helpful:
- Squeeze a lemon in a glass of water and have it sitting on the bathroom or kitchen counter where you'll see it first thing.
- Drink your lemon-water throughout the day to continue the impact.
- At your first meal of the day, get some green veggies into your smoothie or omelet.
- Consider how many more vegetables would you eat, if every time you had lean protein, you added a serving of greens? That can't be a bad thing.

CLEAN AND LEAN PROTEIN

If insulin is the mother of fat storage, glucagon may the father of fat burning. In fact, it has the opposite effect. One critical way to increase this hormone is to eat more protein. This hormone is one that is not included in the chapter that addresses all of the bad boys and divas that may be causing problems with your metabolism. Little is written about glucagon, suggesting not enough is known about it. What you want to know is that it can and does assist in boosting fat burn, as long as your insulin levels are not elevated. You'll read more on that soon.

One of the foods that is most commonly cut out during times of dieting is now the key to losing weight. A woman will say, "I have a hard time getting in all the protein." She'll commit to doing it and agree she feels better doing it, but it is a major shift in thoughts and actions at every meal and snack all day every day.

You really don't want to lose weight. You want to lose, in fact remove, fat. You don't want to find it again. The problem with diets over time, even dieting with exercise, is that a percent of the weight lost is always muscle. In the end, that does not help either your metabolism or your health, and is usually cause for more weight gain in your not-so-distant future. Protein spares muscle, even on low-calorie diets.

If you want to lose weight with less hunger, more satisfaction, and fullness, you want protein. Higher protein diets prevent reduction in energy expenditure that typically accompanies the diet diva. The results are even better when you combine a diet rich in lean protein with physical activity. Your *After 50 Fitness Formula* for weight loss is high protein, plus low glycemic-load foods, plus physical activity, particularly resistance training.

Hormone-free, antibiotic-free, free-range, wild-caught, grass-fed—while it may seem endless, you need to know if these things are true about the foods you put in your system. You are what you eat. You are also what you eat eats. If your food has been fed hormones, then you're eating them. If your food has eaten grasses treated with pesticides, then you're eating them.

Seafood and fish sources of protein may work best if you have a lot of stress. Here's why. Although estrogen levels drop with menopause, you may have hormone trickery going on. Your stress hormone, cortisol, can block progesterone production, which will create a state of estrogen dominance. Estrogen and progesterone should have similar levels. Eliminating red meat, poultry, and dairy temporarily can help. These foods are more likely to contain hormones. It's worth a short break from these foodstuffs to test how you feel. If or when you return to eating these foods, choose organic, hormone, and antibiotic-free meats. If you've wondered if it really matters, the answer is yes.

The controversy about animal versus plant-based protein is not one this book can hope to put to bed. Whether you choose vegan or vegetarianism for spiritual, animal rights, or other reasons, that's your right. No one is attempting to change your mind about that.

There's no question that if you're vegan and consuming 100 percent of your protein from plant-based sources, that it's not all that easy to get the amount of protein that research suggests will help you keep your lean muscle tissue. It's not impossible; it's just harder.

❏ How Much Is Enough?

In the U.S., the current recommendation is for 0.8 grams of protein daily for each kilogram of your body weight, or 0.36 grams per pound. That's about 71 grams a day for the average 196-pound U.S. man, or 60 grams for the average 166-pound U.S. woman. (These are the current average weights in America.) It should be noted that some nutritionists suggest an increased range of up to 1.2 grams per gram of body weight for bodybuilders, as well as for endurance athletes and rapidly growing adolescents. This recommendation is progress.

❑ The Recommended Daily Allowance (RDA)

The RDA has a number of potential obstacles concerning the daily consumption of protein, including the following:

- First, it's not user-friendly. Generally stated in grams of protein recommended for kilograms of your body weight, the mere mathematical dilemma doesn't help you plan your daily intake.
- Second, this total implies that the protein can be taken in at any time. Because there is no breakdown of meals, snacks, or timing, an individual is left to make her own assumptions.
- Third, protein recommendations come in percentages of total daily intake. The recommended range of protein intake is 10 to 35 percent. Many registered dietitians are shifting to see the higher end of the range (i.e., 35 percent) as a better alternative, based on weight-loss research. This situation, however, still presents a math problem. A person needs first to know their desirable daily caloric intake, adhere to it, and do the math for the recommended consumption of protein grams.

People tend to like labels, such as "high-protein," "low-carb," and "low-fat" diets, which can help you organize your thoughts. But, it's relative. You have to ask, *high compared to what?* As such, you can see the dilemma in using the term "high-protein" diet. If you're eating a diet of 10 percent protein now, increasing to 33 percent will be "higher" but not necessarily a "high-protein diet."

It could be said that most Americans currently eat a "low"-protein diet. In fact, such an inference is true of many adults in the second 50. One-third of adults over 50 fail to meet even the current RDA for protein. The assumption is that since they are less active and want to avoid weight gain, they need less protein. The very opposite is true, whether you're 50 or you're 90, and whether you are mildly active, an athlete, or bedridden.

Your lean muscle peaked when you were about 25 years old. Muscle losses each decade range between 3 to 8 percent thereafter. Sexy goes on vacation, and fat moves in. It's not inevitable, unless you ignore your need for protein, snack on low-calorie but high fat-producing foods, and ignore weight training. That's a fat-building formula.

Due to your potential cumulative losses over decades and times of illness, injury, or inactivity, an adequate dietary intake of calories and protein is one of the only ways to overcome impending sarcopenia, the muscle-wasting phenomenon that is largely responsible for the frailty and falls that can affect individuals as they age and that was once thought to be inevitable. It is, but only if you're not getting enough calories, protein, and the right dose of exercise.

Since 2008, there have been whispers in many scientific circles of the need to increase RDAs. It's suggested the current RDA should be renamed the *daily minimum amount* to prevent illness and loss of lean body mass. In fact, the average adult may need more protein for optimal living, a point we'll see that is even truer of older adults, who may not adequately utilize the protein they do eat as their younger cohorts do. Some researchers have bolstered their support for moderately increasing protein consumption beyond the current recommended dietary allowance by adopting a meal-based approach to replace the less-specific daily recommendation.

Research points to a protein threshold (approximately 25 to 30 grams per meal) that allows adequate ingestion of essential amino acids for optimal muscle protein synthesis (MPS). The lower end of the range is sufficient for active adults who better synthesize dietary protein for their muscles. Sedentary adults need the upper range. Read that again. It's not intuitive. Check Appendix B-2 to learn just what 25 to 30 grams of protein looks like.

There are a number of potential factors working against you that can cause you to have to fight for your right to party with muscles, including the following:

- *Age.* Just having another birthday compromises muscle protein synthesis. Muscles break down (catabolism) more easily than they build up (anabolism), as you age.
- *Low-calorie or low-protein diet.* Both cause catabolism. If you cut calories and skimp on protein to lose weight, some of your muscles go bye-bye. On the other hand, fat is loyal. If you dieted in your 30s to fit into your skinny jeans, you didn't do yourself any favors for your chances of fitting into your back-of-the-closet clothes at 55.

This is a good time to talk about you and skinny jeans. What if you can't wear skinny jeans? Skinny jeans and healthy weight might not co-exist for you. This is going to be a rocky road (not the kind found in the freezer) for you, if you can't reshape the six inches between your ears. Whatever media stories you bought into about sexy and skinny being the same thing could keep you trapped. You're stuck inside your head—period. Only 13 percent of women over 50 feel good about their body. The other 87 percent don't just pass on dessert. They don't go to the store, let alone dinner and a movie. Don't pass on life.

- *Physical inactivity.* Not using muscles easily leads to muscle wasting. Physical *activity* can also contribute to muscle loss. Muscles break down before they recover and become stronger. Diligent exercise, without enough calories and protein to overcome the natural breakdown that occurs during exercise, will lead to muscle losses. It doesn't matter if you're active or inactive. You are a victim of catabolism crime. It doesn't discriminate.

❏ Too High for Health?

You may wonder about the health risks of a high-protein diet. The 25 to 30 grams of protein per meal could indeed be much higher than the amount you would calculate for your activity level and body weight using RDAs. It is also much higher than the average intake, based even on that of the heavier average weight of Americans today.

It is in line, however, with research suggesting that RDAs should be boosted by 20 to 30 percent or doubled to achieve weight loss. For many Americans, ingesting 90 grams of protein (3 x 30 grams) daily would be the equivalent of eating a diet of 35 percent of protein. This approach is still within current RDA recommendations.

Minimizing your muscle loss to 15 percent or less is ideal during weight-loss programs. Muscle losses can (and probably have in the past), however, reach levels of 42 to 50 percent of your total weight loss. With this type of loss, the regain of weight that happens for 66 percent of dieters, which inevitably is fat, is almost guaranteed. Your metabolism will drop, due to weight and muscle loss.

If you have a protein quantity concern, it's likely to be about your kidneys. There's no evidence in research that the recommendations here cause any negative effect to the liver and kidneys in apparently healthy adults. If you either have an existing condition or are taking medications, you should absolutely consult with your physician about safety and interactions.

❏ Timing Your Protein and Your Exercise for More Lean, Less Fat

Protein synthesis remains above basal levels up to 48 hours after resistance training (and extended endurance exercise). That factor holds, as long as you eat protein. If you don't, that muscle is cannibalizing itself. Continued elevated intake of protein during this period aids recovery, prevents losses, and enhances gains in lean muscle.

Higher-exercise levels of protein intake are suggested for older adults than for younger adults. You're less efficient at muscle protein synthesis at 50 or 60 than you were at 25. One study, for instance, showed 40 grams of post-resistance exercise protein was most beneficial for older adults, while 25 grams was adequate for younger adults.

Research also recommends specifically that you have a pre-exercise snack of 24 grams protein and a post-exercise snack, within 30 minutes after exercise, of 1:3 or 4 ratio of protein-to-carbohydrate. The carbohydrate, which enhances the protein use, is perfect for replenishing muscle glycogen to enhance recovery. Yes, even when weight loss is your goal, you want to input some simple sugars at the appropriate time. Immediately post-exercise—with protein—is the appropriate time.

Chocolate milk that is dairy or soy fits the ratio. If you're not tolerant of either or have eliminated them temporarily (for whatever reason), a protein powder, mixed in water, almond, or rice milk, will substitute. Don't neglect the carbs at this time. If you have a low-carb protein drink, add half a banana to the shake. You want a snack that is easy to absorb and digest. Nuts with fruit or in a yogurt will also provide carbs and protein. But because they are not as easily digested, they are less on-target with your goal at this post-exercise time period.

About 90 minutes post-exercise, your muscles are ripe for a 25 to 30 grams protein meal. If you have a meal planned post-exercise, you don't have to use the 30-minute post-exercise snack window. You, however, want one or the other. Plan ahead.

❑ Your Weight Loss on Protein

Weight loss studies indicate that even severe calorie-restriction, high-protein diets spare muscle losses. Consume 25 to 30 grams of protein three times a day to spare your lean muscle, while you lose fat. Spreading your protein intake across the day's meals is your best option. Ninety grams total is not the same as 25 to 30 grams at breakfast, lunch, and dinner. The secret to success is in the amount of essential amino acids consumed at one time that help optimize muscle protein synthesis (MPS).

Perhaps, the most compelling reason to include protein in your health plan is the fact that dieters who get plenty of protein tend to stick with it. Compliance is higher for relatively long periods of time. The only way for you to see results long-term is to stick with it. By eating adequate amount of protein, you decrease the need for willpower.

Your body's natural reaction to low-calorie diets is low-energy expenditure. Can you say backfire? That scenario can be avoided by timing your quantity of high-quality protein with the right kind of physical activity.

❑ What if You're Vegetarian?

Getting enough protein from plant-based foods alone is a challenge. Once upon a time, you may have thought getting full before you ate many calories was good. In reality, if you get full before you consume enough protein, your sexy muscles won't be as sexy, but your fat will flourish.

There is an abundance of information suggesting it's relatively easy to get all the protein you need from plants. If you're still a believer of the RDA and think if you get at least 10 percent of your total calories from protein, you'll be fine, you might put stock in that guidance. If you have evidence already that what you're doing is not working, consider a change. If you're gaining weight in the form of unwanted fat, start tracking your current protein intake with the 30-day tracking form that is included in Appendix A-6.

Unrelated to protein, but very important to health and energy, there are a couple supplement needs to consider if you're vegan. Vitamin B12 is only absorbed in reasonable amounts from animal sources of protein. The most absorbable iron, heme iron, comes from animal sources. If you're experiencing fatigue on a diet low in animal protein, these two factors are potentially to blame. Animal food sources are the optimal way to get them in and absorbed, but if that's not your personal preference, seek the advice of your physician about supplementing.

Natural vegan sources of protein limit you. Beans, brown rice, quinoa, nuts, and seeds are good plant sources of protein. Imagine a half-cup each of beans and quinoa. The combination would be potentially very filling. Yet, it's only about 14 grams of protein. You've got a lot of fiber filling you up. If meal after meal, day after day, you fall short of protein, your muscles are likely to suffer.

Going the vegan route, consider adding a plant protein blend of brown rice, hemp, and pea-protein powder supplement to your meals. It's not a bad idea even if you're a meat eater to rotate a whey or soy protein powder out if you rely on them daily. The plant-blend will include all the essential amino acids (2.5 grams of leucine per serving is particularly important) so hard to find in a single plant source of protein. Pumpkin seed protein powder can be stirred into smoothies or soups. Even those vegan powders have only 10 to 20 grams of protein however. Plan carefully. Refer to the Resources section for more information on protein powder supplements.

Meat vs. Vegan

So many of the articles citing studies comparing diets of meat-eaters with vegans include a discussion about the elevated disease and increased risk of early mortality in meat eaters. What's true of those studies and not usually discussed is that much of the meat eaten by subjects was farmed (i.e., fed hormones, antibiotics, and caged). The diet of meat eater included very few fruits and vegetables. Subjects had high levels of stress (perhaps from their diets). Furthermore, their pre-existing risk factors were not taken into consideration. As such, the simple interpretation of whether eating animal protein is good or bad is not simple at all.

❏ The *After 50 Fitness Formula* Protein Facts

- You have a greater need than your younger self for protein.
- Evenly distributed meals of adequate protein throughout the day will boost optimal muscle protein synthesis.
- The basic objective is to shoot for 25 to 30 grams of protein at three meals a day.
- No health risks, and in fact positive health results, were evidenced from higher protein diets, whether using a percentage or grams-per-meal approach when testing apparently healthy subjects. If you have liver or kidney disease, have other pre-existing conditions, or are taking any medications, consult your physician.

- As a "second 50," you are at the greatest risk for ingesting too little protein to reach even the current lowest protein recommendations.
- Exercise, aging, and inadequate nutrition provide an environment for a breakdown of muscle that can be offset by improving your calorie and protein intake.
- Your pre- and post-exercise protein consumption will boost the benefits of exercise in preventing muscle losses (catabolism), as well as in losing fat.
- Animal proteins provide the "high-quality" protein used in most research available to date. If you're vegan or vegetarian, be diligent about achieving the same level of protein containing essential amino acids in your meals.

SUGAR: PUBLIC ENEMY NUMBER ONE

Sugar is everywhere, not just in the obvious desserts and treats. Protein bars, fruit juices, green drinks, fruit-only jam, and fruit itself are laden with sugar. It's the domino effect of eating this "fat-free" sweet that is blamed for overweight and obesity in our country. The higher the sugar loads of your foods, the higher your insulin response that halts fat metabolism and causes more fat storage. Fat cells grow bigger, they're relocated to the belly, and what's worse, sugar is as addicting as any substance.

The average American eats 20 tsps. of sugar a day. Even if you think you don't, chances are it's sneaking into your diet. You're born with a preference for sweet. Just like you develop a higher threshold for sweet the more of it you have, you can reduce your taste for sweetness with patience. You get a new set of taste buds about every 11 days, suggesting that if you slowly decrease your sweet foods, you can retrain your sensitivity so that you enjoy food just as much without the sugar. Pair any food with a fat or something sour to make it seem sweeter. When you eat your vegetables with cheese, broccoli will taste sweeter. When babies are exposed to vegetables first, they enjoy them. Once they're exposed to fruits, the vegetables often don't go down quite as easily. During orientation meetings, new clients often admit that they don't get all their vegetables in. With pride, they'll report that they're better about fruit. You don't say.

Even if you've sworn off desserts, there's a strong chance you're eating more sugar than you realize. Drinking wine on an empty stomach? It's metabolized as sugar. Whatever you eat after drinking the wine is more easily stored as fat. Substituting "natural" sugars for refined? Your body responds the same way. Even artificial sugar may keep you craving the sweet taste. If you really want to bust through this fat trap, you have to make your mind up to defeat cravings that will happen, unless you say no to sugar. It's more addicting than cocaine. You're going to have withdrawals.

Check your salad dressing labels. Balsamic vinegar dressing is made with sugar. Even your favorite ranch may have corn syrup in it. While fruits contribute to your sugar content, so do starchy vegetables like potatoes and corn, as well as white breads, white rice, and pastas. Choose berries and citrus fruits and reduce your intake of sweeter fruits to keep your sugar load lower. The glycemic index (GI) that grades all foods, based on the white potato's score of 100, has been the standard way to track sugar intake.

Glycemic load is a more practical way to apply the GI to your diet, and is easily calculated by multiplying a food's GI (as a percentage) by the number of net carbohydrates in a given serving. JJ Virgin, author of the *Sugar Impact Diet,* has simplified the process of making sense of the real impact of sugar on your body. The GI has limits, since a food is simply ranked on a fixed weight, not on serving size. As a result, carrots, for instance, rate high on GI. Their overall sugar impact, or glycemic load (GL), however, is low. Some comparisons are detailed in the following sidebar.

GI of baked russet potato: 111
GL of baked russet potato: 33

GI of pretzels: 82
GL of pretzels: 16

GI of carrot: 71
GL of carrot: 7.2

GI of sweet potato: 54
GL of sweet potato: 13.1

GI of corn: 62
GL of corn: 20

GI of white rice: 89
GL of white rice: 43

GI of peanuts: 7
GL of peanuts: 0

Just what do you do about your cravings and that sweet tooth? First, stop addressing it like it's a license to have sugar. Second, start checking your labels and removing foods from your diet that have hidden sugars, in addition to the obvious. While you're doing that, try adding lemon to your water. Do you remember that it helps your pH? Sour taste can also help stifle your sweet tooth.

❏ Take the Carbage Out

Nutrition expert Jonny Bowden has told audiences, "Don't eat anything with a barcode." It's nearly impossible today, when even your spinach has a barcode, but it's brilliant. The closer you can come, the better. Choose minimally processed food, bought local and recently alive. Check the ingredients; the fewer the better. The shorter the shelf life of a food you buy, the longer yours will be if you eat it.

This particular moment in your life is a perfect time for a pantry raid. Whatever you do, don't give away your carbage. So, you made the mistake of buying crap before you were educated and committed. No one else, including the homeless or the women's shelter, needs crap either. Throw it where it belongs. Expiration dates long past are a sign to toss. Beyond that, you now know that added sugars, words you can't pronounce, and too long a list of ingredients rob you of health benefits. Start cleaning out now or finish this chapter and then get armed with your garbage bag. If it's in there, you'll eat it. If it's in there, your family will eat it. Are you comfortable with that? Are you comfortable naked in daylight?

Start fresh by trying to eat from as few barcodes as possible at every meal. Consider whether it was recently alive, or if it came wrapped in marketing. Did you get it in the garden, at the farmer's market, or did it come from another country? If it's 20 below and the ground is frozen, your vegetables can be too.

Generally speaking, you should reduce your intake of starchy vegetables, e.g., corn, peas, and white potatoes. Slower absorbed carbohydrates, like sweet potatoes, quinoa, white kidney beans, and steel-cut oats are good carbohydrates that will give you energy for hours, without spiking your blood sugar. Non-starchy cruciferous vegetables can substitute well for pizza-crust ingredients or mashed potatoes. It's a transition, but once you make it, you may love the taste as much as you love the way you feel.

Swaps for Your Favorite Comfort Carbs

- *Buns or wraps—romaine lettuce, endive, or coconut wraps*
- *Mashed potatoes—mashed cauliflower or sweet potato*
- *Noodles—kelp noodles*
- *Pizza crust—cauliflower or zucchini*
- *Rice—cauliflower rice or sweet potatoes*

❏ What Time Is Carb Time?

Timing your carbs is important. It's also not intuitive. Advice to stop eating carbs after 3 p.m. or 4 p.m. is common. That makes sense from a standpoint that you may be less active later in the day, and you don't need calories to sleep. It's not a one-size-fits-all notion, though. It also works in reverse. You help ensure that you'll be less active late in the day, if you give yourself less energy. Your body responds by trying to expend less. If you're on the go all day, you may feel better with a few more (quality) carb calories later. Those late-day carbs are what fuels morning workouts too.

Tame your hormones with the right timing. Cortisol dictates that you need to shift some carbs to your evening meal. If you have signs of cortisol imbalance—you're stressing about something, you have afternoon cravings, or you're having a hard time sleeping—invite a small sweet potato or quinoa to dinner. The carbs can help you offset low cortisol levels that tend to occur late in the day and help you sleep, which can decrease cravings tomorrow.

REPLACE MADE-IN-A-PLANT FOODS WITH PLANT FOODS

Natural plant food, lean protein, and minimally processed foods should be your staples. When you both remove chemicals from additives and preservatives, and add phytochemicals from fresh vegetables and low-sugar fruits, your system will begin to heal from the inside out.

"I can eat anything I want when I exercise." If you've ever been able to say that, you're in the minority. The reality is most people just can't do that and manage their health successfully. The good news is that the more active you become, the more you want to fuel your body well. Overcompensating with food after exercise, because you think you earned it, can derail your results, regardless of your age. If you're often tempted to overeat after exercise, rework your exercise plan. Reduce the duration first. Tons of long, slow exercise, the kind you may have gotten into the habit of doing, can elevate your appetite unnecessarily.

Physical activity is an important part of health. But, it isn't a calorie-burning hall-pass for eating carbage and chemicals. The wrong kind of exercise can increase your desire for sugary foods. Exercise then becomes punishment for the calories. It's a vicious cycle you can't win. You'll have a better chance of enjoying exercise because of the way that you feel from good fuel, instead of only enjoying the results from it after it's over. Joy in movement is the ticket to a long-lasting active life of lean. Whether you choose more exercise or less exercise, physical activity is not optional.

IF IT'S GREEN, IT BOOSTS YOUR LEAN

Phytochemicals feed a lean body and a vibrant skin. They are what your body really craves. They provide vitamins, minerals, and fiber to help you avoid cravings for other things in your diet that sabotage your best health.

If you want the secret to fewer wrinkles or saddlebags, you'll find it faster by trying to include three to six cups of vegetables a day. Shut the door! Six cups of vegetables? It's not as hard as it sounds. What's a day in the life of a leafy green goddess? If you add spinach to a smoothie in the morning, you've already had a cup and a half. Have a salad or soup with veggies at lunch, and you've downed two more cups. If you snack on hummus and crudités, you've added another cup. At dinner, you steam or roast vegetables and fill half of your plate with greens. You're home. Your skin and your belly will both thank you.

FAT IS WHERE SATISFIED IS AT

Contrary to popular belief, recent studies have shown that eating fat does not significantly impact weight or fat gain and that, in some cases, actually speeds up weight loss. Even the consumption of full-fat dairy products (with the exception of those containing probiotics, which boosted losses) had no effect on the weight of the subjects in those studies. Nuts, which are high in mostly monounsaturated fat, were closely associated with weight loss. Topping the list of seemingly slimming foods is (full-fat) yogurt.

Stop. Check in with your response right now. Can you imagine standing in front of the yogurts and reaching for the full-fat yogurt? If there's even the slightest chance you're thinking if you choose the non-fat that you'd lose even more weight, your old habits are messing with you.

It is the fat that increases fullness and satisfaction. Women do some strange math, sometimes. Will non-fat yogurt and a slice of full-fat cheesecake balance out? No! You may be looking for answers in this book, because you've been trying to do math like that for years. The full-fat yogurt may actually curb your craving for the high-sugar cheesecake. Curb your appetite, and curve your body. Eat fat when it counts.

When you increase the amount of fat you eat (applause to you for doing so, since it breaks most of the mental barriers about fat making you fat that you probably picked up along the way), you could unknowingly be causing inflammation. Too strictly adhering to some popular diets can cause your intake of omega 6 fats to be too high in relationship to omega 3 fats. Omega 6 causes inflammation. Omega 3 reduces inflammation. If you're virtuously snacking away on almonds daily, pay attention to this section. You don't want "hot" after 50 to be due to inflamed internal tissues that keeps you chubby and sick.

It's time to get intimate with fat. Not the fat on your belly, back of your arms, or your thighs, but fat in your diet. If your search for optimal health and ideal weight has led you to popular healthy "diets," they may have some flaws.

One big concern about some popular diets is a disproportion of omega 3, 6, and 9 fats, a fact with which most of the experts agree. Wellness authority, Dr. Andrew Weil, first brought awareness of the fact that the ratio of omega 3 to omega 6 fats is not favorable for health. Omega 6 and 9 are already abundant in your diet. Some popular diets, even those adapted as lifestyles, increase the amount of omega 6 you eat.

The problem with inflammation is that you don't see it, and you can be experiencing better well-being and weight improvements without negative problems initially. Internal inflammation—the kind that leads to disease like heart disease and cancer—is the basic issue in this instance.

Omega 3 fats you know as "good" and as something that should be included in your diet. They have an anti-inflammatory response in your body. During the post-exercise period, as well as during times of psychological stress, they aid recovery.

Omega 6, on the other hand, is the inflammatory-causing kind of fat. While you need some omega 6 in your diet, it should be in a specific proportional relationship with omega 3. A ratio of 1:1 or 1:2.1 of omega 6 to omega 3 is recommended by experts, with an equal or heavier amount of omega 3 than 6. The typical American diet is more like 20:1.

Most foods that contain one contain the other. Certain oils and foods contain much higher levels of omega 6, however, and when the overconsumption of those oils and foods are coupled with the underconsumption of omega 3, an imbalance and an inflammatory loop can be created.

Nuts, for instance, are high in omega 6. Snacking on nuts is highly recommended. On the other hand, if you're eating such snacks frequently, or multiple times a day, and without consuming fatty fish or fish oil (high in omega 3) just as regularly, it could be a problem. Another example is oils. Some oils known to you as "healthy," sway too far to the higher omega 6 ratios. The most optimal oils include olive (use at lower temperatures), coconut (best for higher temperatures), avocado, and macadamia.

Omega 3 fats from animal sources may be more optimal than those from plants. As of this writing, most of the benefits of omega 3 fats have been found from EPA and DHA versions of omega 3 that are found in fish. Plant-based ALA omega 3 benefits are less clear. Getting enough of ALA is easier. Vegans and vegetarians may need to supplement their diets. The older you are, in fact, the more you may want to supplement daily with a small dose of fish oil, whether you're vegan or not.

❑ The Best Way to Balance Omega 3 and 6 Fats

Balancing omega 3 and 6 fats is a tricky task. Most experts agree that because these kinds of fats are all "volatile," even the good ones, you don't just want to increase omega 3 to balance sky-high levels of omega 6. You want to both reduce your intake of omega 6 and increase your intake of omega 3. In that regard, there are a couple of steps you can take, including the following:

- Eat fewer foods high in omega 6 and low in omega 3. Don't overdo your intake of nuts and seeds.
- Increase foods that have high omega 3 and low omega 6 content. Increase your consumption of fish and seafood or fish oils, as well as flax and chia seeds. Use coconut, olive, and avocado oils, as well as macadamia oils, when you're cooking or creating salad dressing.

What you can't see, can hurt you. If you're apparently healthy, you may not have any idea that you have internal inflammation. It's not going to cause pain, but it does hurt. It can be creating an environment for disease. It can also be a part of failing weight-loss efforts, even if you're doing everything else right.

❑ New Fat on the Block

Wouldn't it be great, if the fat you ate helped you feel more full and satisfied, *and* burned more calories? There just might be a pot at the end of the rainbow. The fat content in medium-chain triglycerides isn't stored in the body as fat, but instead, it increases the rate at which you burn fat. Score!

Coconut oil is one source of medium-chain fat and why it's winning popularity contests. It's also why you may want to add it to your shopping list. Then, add a tablespoon of it to a smoothie in the morning. Use it to stir-fry your veggies for dinner or as the oil to make your salad dressing. It's available both in liquid and more solid (but liquid at warm temperatures) forms. You can sprinkle raw coconut on cereals or add it to smoothies, too.

❑ More Fat, Less Weight?

If you were ever told that if you feel hungry, you're losing weight, you need to shake that from your idea tree. The truth is that if you went too long between meals, long enough maybe to have your stomach-growling pass, you were probably slowing your metabolism down.

The following three factors are key to long-term weight loss:
• Satiety—feeling of fullness
• Satisfaction—pleasure
• Metabolism—maintenance of lean muscle for more energy expenditure, both at rest and in physical activity

What's missing? Deprivation, hunger, and the need for willpower are not a part of a long-term plan that leads to happiness. If you can't maintain the habits that make you lose weight, there's a big chance you also can't maintain any change that occurs under those conditions.

Fat is a big part of increasing positive feelings about a way of eating you enjoy and will live with for life. Fat doesn't fit into the calorie-controlled diets of the past. Fat, on the other hand, helps you fit into all of the clothes in your closet—with attitude.

FOOD COMBINING HYPE OR HIP?

Contrary to old beliefs about food combining and your body being unable to digest different foods at the same meal, that's not the problem. The question is whether after digestion, foods get stored as fat or not.

Some nutritionists suggest not pairing fats and starches in the same meal (skip the potatoes with your salmon and have broccoli instead), because although fats are neutral, they can exacerbate insulin's fat-storing action.

Having another type of protein with starch would be OK. Cod or chicken, each with less fat than salmon, can be paired with a sweet potato. Chili, with beans and lean meat, will also work. Yet, some experts will warn that if you're not an active person and you're trying to lose weight, the high starch content (up to 70 percent) of beans may be something you want to avoid.

As a vegan, avoiding starches is fairly impossible, if you hope to include protein. The fact that lean and muscular vegan athletes exist suggests that the body is able to adapt to its circumstances.

FIBER FOR SAFE EVACUATION

It's recommended that women 50 or younger consume 25 grams of fiber daily. Daily fiber recommendations for women who are 51 and older drop to 21 grams. It's estimated that most Americans get 15 grams of fiber daily. If you're an active woman over 50, or you're yearning for that title, chances are more fiber is going to keep you moving better inside and out.

Some experts in weight loss and the toxic effects of environment and food suggest that you need significantly more fiber in your diet. Toxins are stored in the fat. If you have 20 pounds or more to lose, significantly increasing your fiber intake may help you to remove toxins as they're released from fat. Promoting this more rapid evacuation of toxins will help you feel better, as you lose weight, by removing the harmful toxins faster.

The first step to optimal fiber is knowing your current daily fiber intake. Read labels. Use Google search. Track your fiber count using the 30-day form that is included in Appendix A-6. Increase your intake of fiber by five grams a day for a week at a time, until you at least meet the minimum. The gradual increase, along with a corresponding increase in your intake of water, will help your system avoid the undesirable gas, bloating, or constipation that you might experience otherwise.

If you have significant weight to lose, nutritionists recommend consuming 35 to 50 grams of fiber a day. As you begin to focus on green leafy and cruciferous vegetables, berries, and nuts and seeds, you'll find it easy to get more fiber into your day.

Flax and chia, along with rice bran, are easy ways to add fiber power to smoothies, salads, and veggies. Real food is better than a fiber supplement.

WHAT'S THE CATCH?

It's sounding too good to be true. Are you thinking that? What do you have to eliminate? Are you waiting for that other shoe to drop? It's a safe bet that your past random acts of dieting and exercise haven't worked, if you picked up this book. Or maybe, you want to keep things going on the right path and avoid detours.

Your usual diet habits can be wrecking your results, without you knowing it. If you're at least 50, you've been raised to believe that dairy, wheat, and grains are a part of good health. Do you remember 4-4-3-2 from back in the day? Grains and dairy foods were the foundation for a good diet. Those thoughts are hard to give up. They may in fact be the brick wall you're hitting. For many women, these foods cause internal inflammation. In combination with antibiotics, illness, and over-the-counter meds, they can be a stomach bomb.

There are plenty of books available on the market, including *Wheat Belly* and *Grain Brain* (refer to Appendix B-6 for details), that give you far greater insight than this brief synopsis. The cliff notes are basically that the quality of those foods at the present time, as well as your possible too frequent consumption of them in the past, paired with a far greater toxic environment than generations past had, could mean that these foods are causing problems for you. You may need to heal your inflammation.

We can't see it like an open wound, so we ignore it. Women tend to think that there's something wrong with them or that they don't have time to stop and figure it out. You probably wrestle with decades of old information, playing like an 8-track in your head, when you're staring at food in the grocery store. If you have gas, bloating, or unexplained weight gain or lethargy, you shouldn't just accept it as normal.

An entire chapter (#7) of this book is devoted to the subject of rest and recovery. In contrast, the current chapter (#3) addresses the other R&R, referred to by many holistic-health practitioners as an elimination diet—remove and reintroduce. You go without the most highly targeted trouble foods for a time and then reintroduce them. You learn a lot about your response to foods by doing that. In fact, it's really one of the only ways to know, once and for all, how foods affect you, at least at the present time. Food sensitivities, unlike allergies, don't cause an immediate severe reaction. That's what makes them hard to detect. Test; don't guess. A food allergy test can still reveal foods that might trigger a milder response for you. Ask your physician about testing.

The following is the hit list of foods that could be keeping you from your best self. While the list isn't all-inclusive, it does include the most common offenders:
- Sugar
- Dairy
- Wheat/gluten
- Meat
- Soy
- Caffeine

If you've got great energy, great digestion, and feel good, there may be no reason to do this step. If what you're doing is not working, and you're ready to take the elimination test, the following tips can help you prepare:
- Plan your meals and snacks, so you are not slashing calories.
- Include plenty of protein during your elimination period.
- Commit to one to three weeks for each food you remove, one at a time.
- Consider reducing the amount of exercise you engage in during this time. While you absolutely can be active, just don't plan your elimination test during preparation for a marathon. Honor your energy level.
- Don't put it off until the timing is perfect. It will never be. Just start. The elimination-diet police are not coming if you mess up once or twice.
- Set up your environment, so you have the right things on hand, so that doing the right thing is relatively easy.

- Remember that caffeine can be a challenging issue for you, if you like your java. If you have two or fewer cups of coffee a day, and you're done by 10 a.m., there's less worry. If you're a pot-on all day gal, or you reach for soda later in the day, you need to can it literally. Cut back to two cups early in the day. If you're not feeling better after your food elimination and reintroduction process, try to eliminate your consumption of caffeine completely. If you have a lot of stress, or a lack of sleep, and/or anxiety is a real challenge, caffeine control could be a big part of helping you feel better. You might have to feel worse first.

Periodically, you may find that stress or old habits start causing digestive problems, and you need to repeat the elimination diet. Periods of illness, taking medications, or experiencing big stressors can change your gut's reaction to foods. While you're doing the elimination diet, your gut gets a chance to heal. As a result, what bothers you at the present time may eventually be OK again. Some women find introducing small amounts of certain trigger foods is fine, while more can get them into trouble. Other women find leaving a trigger food out altogether is what it takes to feel their best. An elimination diet journal is included in Appendix A-3. Never forget that you're the expert on how your body responds.

If you begin to listen to your body and stop settling for discomfort, irritating gas, or digestive problems, you'll know when it's time to clean the slate again. A lot of so-called "cleanses" are out there that are drastic and rob you of nutrients. This whole-food approach doesn't involve cutting calories and only temporarily removes potential irritants, until you reintroduce them. It's like taking your furniture out to polish the floors. You move it back in when everything is ready. You might discover that you need new blinds. Or, you might just love what's happened with the right setting in place, making everything seem new again.

A DAY IN THE DIET OF A LEANER MORE ENERGETIC YOU

Breakfast seems to be the biggest hurdle for most women. Not just because it's the first meal of the day, but also because you may be in the habit of skipping it. It's a sign that either you eat later in the evening, or your level of metabolism is sluggish.

Maybe you like breakfast, and just can't figure out what to eat. You might have started off in life with a regular dose of sugar from a box. You know that's not going to work. You went through the bagel phase and gained weight eating that low fat disc. Now you're unsure. Eggs? Yogurt? Smoothie? Will a protein bar on the way out the door work? (Refer to the barcode statement earlier.)

If you're resistant to breakfast, nail down the reason. Are you really that short on time? There are options that could take from seconds to minutes at most. You could prepare it in advance and eat or drink all or part of it on the way. Are you not hungry? Or, like many women, are you still thinking if you start "on empty," that you'll eat fewer calories all day and lose weight as a result?

That sluggish morning appetite is a sign. Your metabolism needs a boost. You can do that by changing habits on both ends of bedtime. Start with breakfast. Get yourself adapted by starting small. On the flip side, make sure you're leaving two to three hours after your evening meal before bed.

Start with a protein drink. Avoid buying a commercially made ready-for-you option and make your own. If your excuse is you don't have the five minutes to dump and blend it in the morning, you can make it the night before and refrigerate it. With a simple formula, you have infinite options. You'll find a few recipes in Appendix B-3 to get you started.

Lunch and dinner are similar in content, with a few more carbohydrates skewed to your evening meal. If you just had a mild panic attack, because you've been told to limit carbs after three or four in the afternoon, you'll have to trust me. Most women working their way through menopause experience stress, either from weight gain, uncomfortable flashes, or life itself. Stress often causes poor sleep quality or quantity. Afternoon energy drain and cravings are common if your sleep is suffering. If that's you, then a few more quality carbs in the evening can help you relax and sleep better. You'll reduce cravings and not experience those lows in the afternoon.

Protein and lighter carb content at lunch will help you stay alert and focused, as well as head cravings off at the pass. A light protein-rich lunch and a planned early-to-mid-afternoon snack have helped a lot of women boost their energy levels and avoid vending machine temptations.

Your body likes routine. Think about the times when you color outside the lines. How do you really feel when you work your way from one holiday buffet to the next? What do you want to do after a huge Thanksgiving Day meal? When you return from vacation, do you ever need a vacation to recover? Your body has a hard time processing a lot of food at once. It also has a hard time processing a lot of new-to-you foods at once.

Women know intuitively that they do better with routine. Listen to conversations. They say things like, *"I get into a rut." "I tend to eat the same things over and over."*

The situation isn't all bad! You can have a smoothie for breakfast, a salad and soup for lunch, and protein and vegetables for dinner seven days a week and still get a lot of variety. Change up the kind of protein powder, greens, fruit, and fat in your smoothies. Vary the kind of protein and veggies you add to your salad. Prepare various protein options on the grill, or bake or stir-fry instead. Switch up your spices. The next section of this chapter provides a simple menu template of options. Choose what works best for you. The point is, get one. If you like a breakfast you can sink your teeth into, leave the smoothies for your pre- or post-exercise snack. If a salad just doesn't do it for you at lunch, opt for something else.

There is nothing wrong with breaking the rules. Leftovers from the night before at breakfast are fine. Keep in mind that routine rocks. Your body responds well to a pattern of eating. You may notice that when you travel, either because the food fare or the schedule is so different, your digestion suffers a little. A little flexibility helps nutrient variety and your satisfaction. If smoothies appeal to you, use the smoothie formula in Appendix B-3 and get creative. If you love fresh salads, change up the veggies and the lean protein you add.

Snack according to your needs. Three to four hours between meals is good timing. If you find you're hungry more frequently, look at your meals and make sure you have adequate protein and fiber, as well as healthy fat in your meals. If you have more time between meals due to your schedule, snacks may be really important for you. If you find you do best with smaller and more frequent meals, be conscious of quality and content.

Breakfast:

- *Protein shake formula: (liquid, protein powder, fat, greens, berries, ice)*
- *Eggs: scrambled, omelet, burrito with veggies on gluten-free tortilla*
- *Steel cut oats with protein, nuts, berries, cinnamon*

Lunch:

- *Lean protein: grilled, baked, poached, protein shake*
- *Creamy non-dairy or broth-based soup*
- *Vegetables: fresh salad, grilled, crudités*
- *Wrap: non-gluten, sprouted, lettuce*

Dinner:

- *Lean protein: grilled, baked, roasted*
- *Non-starchy vegetables: fresh salad, steamed, roasted, sautéed*
- *Slowly absorbed carbohydrate: quinoa, sweet potato, tortilla*

Snacks:

- *Boiled eggs*
- *Hummus with fresh veggies*
- *Half a simple protein shake ("milk" with protein powder)*
- *Mixed nuts or seeds*
- *Chia "pudding"*

PRE- AND PROBIOTICS: LIVE AND ACTIVE CULTURES

Trusting your gut instinct gets easier at midlife, but trusting that your gut is working right gets harder. If you've got a history of taking antibiotics or over-the-counter medications, or you've suffered illness and high levels of stress, chances are your gut health may not be optimally helping you with your sexy-after-50 mission. Antibiotics destroy bacteria-causing illness, but, unfortunately, they also destroy the good bacteria that you need at the same time.

Probiotics and prebiotics can help improve the "good" bugs in your gut and reduce or eliminate the "bad" bugs. Probiotics introduce good bacteria into the gut. Prebiotics fertilize the good bacteria already there. During your elimination diet, you may further benefit by adding pre/probiotics to help heal your gut.

For probiotics to have any beneficial effects, they need to reach the intestine alive and in sufficient numbers. Some products contain cultures in insignificant amounts—or may have, at some point, contained cultures that have since been destroyed during the manufacturing process. For a product to claim it has live and active cultures, it needs to show it has more than 100 million bacteria per gram at the time of manufacture. Fermented foods, including tempeh, miso, sauerkraut, and kombucha, contain microorganisms that may not only benefit gut health, but also enhance appetite-suppressing hormones.

❑ Culture Count

Ingesting one billion CFUs (colony-forming units) per day is helpful for simply maintaining gut health. As such, you should ingest 10 billion CFUs per day, if you're trying to reduce the severity of a gastrointestinal illness.

❑ Culture Specificity

Because some probiotics work best for specific illnesses, variety is better. Look for one that lists multiple culture strains.

❑ Pills or Food?

During times of stress—increased exercise, family/work pressures, illness—it might be prudent to increase your consumption of beneficial bacteria. Accordingly, you may need to supplement your diet with pills or with specialty probiotic "shots," such as Yakult, DanActive, or Good Belly Shots. Bacteria can also be concentrated and packaged into pills or tablets for an even greater concentration of CFUs. Because strains and strain count vary greatly, as does the recommended dosage, check labels carefully.

You make hundreds of decisions about food every day. Your choices decide your health, energy, and weight. Isn't it time to start enjoying more good food, so you can feel good more?

Celebrity Nutrition and Fitness Expert JJ Virgin

❏ Why Most Plans Miss the Bigger Sugar-Impact Picture

As experts and newer studies confirm that a high-sugar impact diet creates obesity and other devastating health repercussions, manufacturers have devised new ways to give unhealthy foods a health halo. You've seen the hyperbolic claims on packaged foods, such as *low glycemic index, high-fiber, fructose free*, etc.

Likewise, a number of popular diet plans focus exclusively on the glycemic index or eating nutrient-dense foods. While these perspectives become perfectly legitimate, focusing on one aspect often overlooks others that dramatically affect a food's sugar impact.

In that regard, a review of the strengths and limitations of the following four ways to measure a food's sugar impact can be helpful:

- *Glycemic index or load.* The glycemic index (GI) measures how a food impacts your blood sugar levels. Pure glucose is ranked highest at 100, while all other foods are measured accordingly. The higher its glycemic rating, the greater the effect a food will have on your blood sugar. Because GI doesn't account for quantity, researchers developed the glycemic load (GL), a measure that combines the glycemic index with serving size.

  If you're not into math, the situation can become confusing. Besides, you don't eat foods in isolation. Determining how foods raise blood sugar in different combinations becomes virtually impossible. GL also makes fructose look like an angel, since fructose doesn't raise blood sugar.

- *Fructose.* Critics like Dr. Robert Lustig consider fructose the most metabolically damaging sugar. Among its problems, an excessive consumption of fructose creates insulin resistance, raises triglycerides, increases your risk for numerous diseases, like Type 2 diabetes and heart disease, and eventually finds a nice home around your midsection.

  Fructose also doesn't activate insulin or leptin, the hunger hormone that tells your brain to stop eating. Because both hormones impact satiety levels, you can easily overeat fructose without your brain getting the "halt" message.

  By fructose, I mean high-fructose corn syrup and fructose-sweetened processed foods. Naturally occurring fructose in whole foods, like fruit and vegetables comes intertwined with fiber and nutrients, which slows fructose's absorption. Because processed, fructose-containing Frankenfoods lack those nutrients and fiber, fructose makes a beeline towards your liver, which has a field day making fat.

Well aware that you've become nutritionally savvier, manufacturers now boast "no high-fructose corn syrup" to somehow imply a healthier food. Don't fall for it. Turn the label over, and you'll likely find another sugar listed among the ingredients. Keep in mind that over 57 names for sugar exist!

• *Nutrient density.* Some eating plans develop intricate charts that rank foods according to their nutrient density, which accounts for vitamins, mineral, phytonutrients, and other compounds in that food. Such plans don't always address the relevant issues. For example, a cup of blueberries contains about 15 grams of sugar. Yet, thanks to nutrients and fiber, berries create a low GL, providing a slow, steady rise in blood sugar that won't trigger a dramatic insulin response.

Because nutrients in nature's foods change the way your body deals with sugar, even a higher-GL tuber or higher-fructose fruit creates less of a sugar impact. Getting 15 grams of sugar from blueberries or a sweet potato creates a totally different effect than getting 15 grams from a granola bar.

Still, eating too many nutrient-dense foods can still deliver a big glycemic and fructose load. Nutrient-density plans also often undervalue protein and fat, which often rank lower in micronutrient amounts, but provide numerous other healthy benefits.

• *Fiber.* Fiber is a fierce secret weapon for balancing your blood sugar and helping you break free from the vice grip of sugar. Knowing its health glow, manufacturers have created fiber-enhanced cookies and other high-sugar impact foods. Furthermore, most diet plans focus exclusively on meeting a certain fiber quota.

While it can indeed buffer a food's sugar impact, adding fiber does not suddenly make a cookie healthy, and a high-fiber diet can still remain a high-sugar impact diet.

❑ Looking at the Bigger Picture

You can see how glycemic load, fructose, nutrient density, and fiber play a role in a food's sugar impact and therefore its healthiness, yet each measure contains limitations. In my book, *Sugar Impact Diet,* I look at all four criteria to determine which foods have the lowest sugar impact. Many folks, unknowingly, have become sugar addicts, and you'll become shocked concerning what "healthy" foods often contain hidden sugars.

Rather than ask you to eliminate these higher-sugar impact foods, on this plan, you gradually taper and transition to a lower-sugar impact plan that helps you burn fat, boost your health, and look and feel your best.

Maybe, you've done a very low-carb or sugar-elimination diet and suffered withdrawal, cravings, and other misery. That's why I created the Sugar Impact Diet. You get fast, lasting fat loss and numerous other benefits of going low-sugar impact without deprivation. With this plan, you'll forever crush sugar addiction, without any drawbacks.

As more studies confirm its detrimental health impact, have you become more aware about how much sugar you consume? Share your story on my website or on my Facebook fan page.

Celebrity nutrition and fitness expert JJ Virgin helps clients lose weight fast by breaking free from food intolerances and crushing their sugar cravings. She is author of New York Times *bestsellers* The Virgin Diet: Drop 7 Foods, Lose 7 Pounds, Just 7 Days; The Virgin Diet Cookbook: 150 Easy and Delicious Recipes to Lose Weight and Feel Better Fast; *and* The Sugar Impact Diet: Drop 7 Hidden Sugars, Lose up to 10 Pounds, Just 2 Weeks. *JJ is also a frequent blogger at Huffington Post, Mind Body Green, and other outlets, as well as a popular guest on TV, radio, and in magazines. Learn more at www.jjvirgin.com.*

We don't become inactive because of age. We age because of inactivity.

CHAPTER 4 ——————————————————
Movement Matters

You were meant to move. Contemporary life is filled with opportunities to be sedentary. Sitting is the new smoking. It's become one of the biggest risk factors in existence. Yet, it's controllable.

If you're not physically active at the present time, your reasons probably include a lack of time, being injured, or a lack of motivation. Your obstacle could be intimidation or discomfort. On the other hand, you'll get sick and die sooner if you don't get physical activity. That's intimidating and uncomfortable. Motivated yet? You'll have less sex, less sleep, earn less, be less productive, and be more likely to be depressed and have one of 80 of the most common diseases if you don't. Motivated now?

If you're reading this book, you're thinking about it. You can exercise less than you think you have to and get good results. If you already like exercise but aren't getting results you want, the sections in this chapter are going to identify the highest priority activities for you. Even if you have a lot of time, you only have so much energy. If you waste it on doing things that don't give you a good return on investment (ROI) in life, you could push yourself farther from your goals instead of moving closer to them.

Exercise with purpose and intention will change your results completely. You want to move away from doing more of the same exercise to doing less. The key, however, is to perform the right exercise. If you're exercising without results, you could be following a belly-fat formula, instead of a flat-belly formula. Oops.

This chapter is relatively long. There are two major elements addressed. They're both covered in the same chapter, because it isn't an either/or option. Both resistance training and cardiovascular exercise should make the A-list for your exercise party. Initially, the chapter considers resistance training and then moves into cardio training. Yes, you need flexibility and mobility. No, you won't find extensive information about it in this book. Don't let that give you the impression that it's any less valuable either for staying safe or, indirectly, for weight loss.

> *I love to see a young girl go out and grab the world by the lapels.*
> *Life's a bitch. You've got to go out and kick ass.*
>
> —Maya Angelou

PART I: STRENGTH TRAINING

WEIGHT LIFTING FOR WEIGHT LOSS

Aerobic activity could make you fat. A study in the *Journal of Strength and Conditioning Research* had 81 previously sedentary premenopausal women walk 30 minutes, three times a week, without changing their diet. Ultimately, the subjects showed no real-weight or fat-mass losses overall. Fifty-five of the 81 women, however, were subsequently labeled as compensators and actually *gained* fat during the 12-week study. Typically, this is not a desired outcome.

Hypothetically, through diet and maybe exercise, you lose weight. If a large percent of that weight is lean muscle, your metabolism will slow. As a result, the rate that you burn calories at rest and doing every other little thing all day will decrease. This situation will set you up for weight gain in the future. Unfortunately, it's like a two-for-one. You don't just gain back what you lost. You get back more.

The only way to offset your newly slowed level of metabolism is to exercise more and eat less. In fact, it's well known that successful weight-maintenance programs include engaging in more activity than do basic weight-loss programs. Forever. Your ever-plummeting metabolism will make you tired and still require fewer and fewer calories. Typically, women both diet and exercise diligently for a short time and then end it and hope that everything works out for them. That's a formula for weight cycling up every time it happens.

There's a better way not to "weigh less" but to weigh ideal, while looking like you weigh less. You can stop being a slave to the scale and start to focus on your health and your happiness. You shouldn't have to check with the scale in the morning to find out if you're happy. Stinky shoes and too much laundry are a better gage.

If you must measure something, measure your inches and your ability to lift a specific amount of weight. The blessing of strength training for a woman with weight to lose is that you will be more successful from the beginning than any time you've ever started an aerobic exercise regimen.

Your *After 50 Fitness Formula* includes a nutrient-rich, satisfying diet, proper aerobic activity, and a good dose of the proper resistance training. While dieting alone may result in weight loss, temporarily, the weight lost, however, tends to be muscle.

THE DOWNSIDE OF WEIGHT TRAINING

If you're a scale slave, there is bad news. Resistance training will blunt your weight loss. A 150 pound woman who strength trains however is more likely to wear a smaller pair of pants than a 150 pound woman who doesn't. Proportions will change like they will not with aerobic-only exercise. Despite the aforementioned study, you could lose weight and get slimmer, temporarily with aerobic-only exercise, if you're not overeating. The results of such an approach will make you skinny-fat. Numerous studies have found, however that you will lose both strength and bone density, if you only do endurance exercise. Lean, light, and fragile is not a good combination.

Osteoporosis and osteopenia are conditions that are characterized by a level of low bone density that puts you at greater risk for fractures. Sarcopenia is loss of lean-muscle tissue associated with aging. While it's not inevitable, it is more probable if you don't lift and eat in favor of muscle. Dynapenia is a loss of muscle strength with aging. Sarcopenia and dynapenia set you up for risk of falling. Osteoporosis and osteopenia, on the other hand, set you up for fractures if you do fall.

At 50, you may be overconfident about your risk of falling. Yet, even your little-known calf muscles predispose you for falls. At middle age, a woman's fall risk that is associated with weak soleus muscles increases. The soleus is the calf muscle underneath the larger gastrocnemius muscle. One of the only ways to develop this particular muscle is to perform seated heel raises (all factors considered, a relatively easy exercise to perform).

The key point to remember is that your current habits determine what happens both at the present time and in future decades. If your muscles go bye-bye, you don't get them back easily. It's not impossible. The deck is just stacked against you.

Once you have passed age 35, strength training becomes truly indispensable for maintaining muscle mass—along with consuming the proper amount of protein and adhering to the right post-workout nutrition habits. If that ship has been departing without you, it's time to reevaluate your exercise routine and put weight training on the A-list in your post-50 party plans.

The irony of the strength training is the attendant gender bias. Men who exercise tend to spend more time lifting. Women who exercise tend to find aerobic activity more appealing. On the other hand, all factors considered, women need strength training more than men. Overall, they're smaller, weigh less, and when they lose estrogen, they lose bone at an even faster rate. Plus, they're more likely to live longer, all the while losing little breadcrumbs of bone along the way. As such, weight rooms should be designed to appeal to women 35 and over, particularly those 50 and over.

As a woman, you should find a gym that feels comfortable or make one at home. Your first rodeo with weight training might be a group-fitness class. It's a natural, if you're already comfortable in such an environment. While it may potentially be a good introduction to weight training, you shouldn't hang your weight gloves on it. Group strength training classes, with their high repetitions, won't help you lose fat or gain lean muscle. *High repetitions* is defined as anything that you can do 15 or more times. Performing multiple sets of higher reps (at lower weight) will not have the same effect on fat, bones, or muscle, as will doing sets of lower reps (with higher weight).

GROUP-FITNESS CLASSES FAIL THE BONE DENSITY TEST

A recent study involving one of the most popular branded group-strength classes found that participants slowed bone mineral density (BMD) losses *only* at the lumbar spine. In other words, a weight training regimen of performing high repetitions with low weight won't otherwise have a positive impact your hip or total bone density. Is it a good starting point? Yes. Everyone should start with low weight and focus on technique for several weeks, if not months. Yet, a personalized program with individual attention, if you need it, will help you load your body in a way that increases your level of lean muscle, increases the amount of fat loss, and improves your BMD. If you haven't a clue about what good form is or where to begin, consult with a trainer one-on-one, instead of standing in the back of a crowded room.

Women underestimate the amount of weight that they can lift so much that many don't even meet minimum weight requirements for muscle endurance. A fear of injury is valid. You don't want to start with a heavy load. You should build up to it. Get help. You can't afford a trainer? Can you afford an injury or a fracture? Paying for even one or two sessions with a trainer could be priceless. In this day and age, you can record your session video or audio and have that training resource to refer to for months.

One relatively large study found that women's self-selected weights tend to gravitate toward 40 percent of a one-repetition maximum (1 RM). For fat free mass (FFM) and bone mineral density (BMD) increases, that's simply not enough. You need to overload your systems to achieve change. The recommended minimum level of resistance is approximately 60 percent of your 1 RM, or about as much as would permit you to perform 15 repetitions of the exercise. In that regard, the optimal range for FFM and BMD is 80 percent, or 10 repetitions. As such, if you can perform 25 repetitions with a weight, it is not helping you reach your goals. Lifting a lighter weight more times does not have the desired effect on either your level of metabolism or your bones.

An informal poll of 20, 000 women, age 50 and older, asked their thoughts about strength training. The majority thought strength training was optional. The majority also list weight loss or weight management as their number one objective with regard to exercising. They aren't connecting the dots. Are you? Poll respondents who chose strength training let their personal preference, or a fitness instructor's preference, for a particular training tool, e.g., body weight, tubing, dumbbells, or machines, dictate what type of weight training they actually did.

WHAT'S WRONG WITH BODY WEIGHT TRAINING?

Certainly, body weight training is better than nothing. If you can handle your body's weight to perform an exercise more than 10 times, however, you're not loading those bones and muscles enough to create positive change. Body weight exercises can elevate your heart rate. They're also fairly convenient to do. In addition, for corrective exercise, they may be your best option. Once you've built up beyond the point where you can do 15 repetitions of any exercise with your body weight, while it might help you tone or define your musculature, it will not contribute as much to your long-term lean slim self. If you have limited time to exercise, the most ROI on your investment of time and energy is from the heaviest weight you can properly handle.

WHEN YOU KNOW YOUR GOALS, YOU KNOW WHAT TO DO

A number of benefits exist from a variety of types of strength training. The ability to rise from a chair, for example, or achieve an enhanced level of metabolism can result from performing a weight training regimen of lifting 70 to 80 percent of your 1 RM. That's lifting 10 to 12 repetitions of the exercise before the weight gets too heavy to properly perform the exercise. This load also has the most positive effect on your BMD. It also has the most potential to boost your level of metabolism for hours after you've wiped the glow from your face.

For some women who feel they're gaining fat by the minute, weight lifting is counterintuitive. You may have a disconnect between the frustrating fat you've gained, on one hand, and the need to lift weight to create more muscle, on the other. In fact, they are potentially one and the same problem. You've lost enough muscle that even without gaining fat, you are fatter.

The following is the sales pitch for weight training in a nutshell. What helps your bones will help prevent body-fat gains, improve your level of body composition (by lean muscle gain and reductions in body fat), and improve your appearance, as well as your proportions. Weight training will increase your overall expenditure of energy (from your post-exercise consumption of oxygen to engaging in an increased level of activity in your life), and decrease your risk of falls and injury. Is weight training looking pretty sexy?

Because so many women have a fear of bulking (more on that soon), a number of instructors and trainers will encourage women to use small weights when training, suggesting that their exercise regimen doesn't have to be "bodybuilding." Honestly, this advice perpetuates your problem. Two- and five-pound weights, unless that is truly all you can lift at least 10 times at the present time, will not change your body composition, whether you want to lose fat or whether you're frail. To lose body fat and help prevent frailty, you need to lift 80 percent of your peak level of strength in order to get lean muscle mass. It can also be helpful for you to better understand the metabolic conundrum of *sarcobesity*, i.e., being both overweight and having too little muscle, a topic that will be covered later in this chapter.

Lifting with power at 60 percent (15- to 20-repetition range) of your 1 RM results in greater energy expenditure than performing slow contractions at either 60 percent or 80 percent of 1 RM. Lifting to develop your power or lifting with power isn't the same as "powerlifting," an activity performed by bodybuilders or competitive lifters—an undertaking that involves performing a specific set of exercises.

Using power refers to performing a lift rapidly and then safely lowering the weight slowly at a 1:4 ratio. Besides being high in energy expenditure during exercise, this approach saves your fast-twitch fibers. Because life involves certain motor skills, you should keep in mind that your fast-twitch fibers can be important for living the life you want, from busting a move in Zumba to preventing falls. You lose your fast-twitch fibers twice as fast as you lose your slow-twitch fibers as you age.

Life is a power sport. From opening the peanut butter jar to hefting grandchildren into your arms to pushing out of a chair, you need strength with speed. In essence, that attribute defines power. On occasion, you've probably been instructed to slow down when you perform strength training. While beneficial in some instances, you also need to apply some speed-of-life movement on a regular basis. One of your greatest needs for power with heavy loads occurs during a fall. You're going to rapidly have to load one of your legs in order to prevent tripping, when you go up a curb and misjudge the height. Maybe, you're navigating a new set of bifocals or are sleep-deprived, carrying the groceries, while juggling your key in the other hand. You either have that power, or you don't.

With all the pros about heavier weight, don't ignore those lighter levels of resistance. Using at 40 percent of your 1 RM, you're typically able to do 28 to 30 repetitions. This kind of exercise not only benefits your gait, it also helps prevent some of your smaller muscles from being lazy or leading to a sense of imbalance. Preventing senior shuffle could be the last thing you're considering, if you're thinking about losing belly fat. Yet, keeping yourself pain-free and with optimal movement patterns is key to you being able to move enough to lose.

You don't have to be 90 and frail for fall situations to occur. It could happen tomorrow. You don't want to ever have to use your power for this purpose, but like insurance, you will be glad it's there if you do. Meanwhile, your tee-shot, your ability to swing grandchildren around, and your capacity to power your bike up the hill so someone can eat your dust are going to blossom.

So, how do you assess your current strength training program or design one that works? If you're seeking a specific result, you need a specific solution. That's not always what you get with the myriad of fitness videos, trainers, and boot camps, all vying for your attention at any given moment. If you selected a video because of the celebrity endorsing it, and you're using it because you like it, that's a small step in the right direction. You should like it. On the other hand, hopefully, the program you selected was because it fit your need for lifting both heavy and light weights, as well as for using power. Not surprisingly, you'll like your program more, if it gets the right results.

Your options aren't really all as optional as you might think. Every 50-plus woman needs some heavy lifting. Every 50-plus woman needs some power, and every 50-plus woman needs functional exercise with light resistance. The issue is how much of each? The ratio of exactly what you need of each element varies with your needs + goals formula. It's an if-this, then-that solution.

First, you want to define heavy, power, or moderate weight, as well as low-weight, repetition ranges. Each of them contributes to your optimal function. That's the take-away point in this instance. "Functional exercise" isn't a category all its own that refers to exercises that are better than others. All exercises are potentially functional, and all weight loads are functional. The question to ask is, *what's functional for you?* Start with purpose. Your new mantra is to perform no more random acts of strength training.

By age 50, you may have an injury or a "niggle." It may mean your "heavy" is limited by a particular joint or condition. "Within your limits" is the unspoken, but all-important, rule to every exercise guideline you read. One problem joint, though, doesn't have to exclude everything. If you have a shoulder issue, for instance, it may keep you from pushing heavy or pressing overhead. Potentially, you can still include heavy pulling, such as performing a rowing exercise, to optimize your metabolism. If you have osteoporosis or fibromyalgia, you need to work safely, as well as progressively, i.e., gradually increase load.

FATIGUE IS GOOD, FAILURE IS UNNECESSARY

Reaching temporary muscular fatigue is a sign that you've overloaded the muscles sufficiently to get stronger, provided you rest enough between exercise sessions. You can reach fatigue with each set. If your goal, for instance, is to perform 10 repetitions of a given exercise, you should select a weight that allows you to have good form and posture through all 10 repetitions. At that point, however, you should begin to feel that you can't maintain the proper form for doing the exercise any longer. *Failure* is complete inability to properly lift the weight one more time. You don't have to get to the point of failure during your lifting regimen. Doing so certainly doesn't increase your progress, but it absolutely does increase your risk of injury.

Heavy is weight that you can't lift more than 10 to 12 times. Sometimes, you have to lift furniture that you'd only like to have to move once, until someone says, *"no, no, over there would be better."* That's heavy. Heavy weight training is the kind of work that helps you get out of a chair. Traditional exercises help you do it, squats and leg presses, for example. Do you agree getting out of the chair is pretty functional? You don't want to wait until you're stuck in the chair to start avoiding getting up. That's exactly what happens with some older adults. Now is the time for you to prepare for your upcoming decades.

Power movements are done a little faster and at either a heavy (80 percent of 1 RM) or a lower weight (60 percent 1 RM max). As a rule, you can perform power movements about 15 to 20 times. Performing repetitions with power involves a more rapid lifting (one count) and a slower lowering (four counts) sequence. While this protocol is best undertaken with cables or air-compression machines for safety, when they're not available, machines and free weights can be used. Tubing and bands can be used, as long as the resistance allows the right rep range.

Light resistance loads are 40 percent of your maximum weight lifted, which translates into a repetition range of 28 to 30. Side-stepping with light resistance tubing, water exercises, and walking with bands all fall into this category. These are the things that help you with gait and corrective movements that help you align and move better with less pain. Maximal power can be generated with heavy or power loads, as well as with light weights. The trick with a light weight is to not allow momentum to take over.

If you want optimal body composition, function, and aging benefits, you need all of the aforementioned options. What percentage of each option do you need? Just how do you piece together your weight-training puzzle?

Consider three different goals. Weight loss, bone density, and fall reduction, and performance in sports or the sport of life are the most common goals of women in their second 50. Of the three—weight loss, bone density, and performance—the most significant is weight loss. If you raised your hand for all three, that's OK too.

If weight loss is your primary goal, remember the disclaimer: weight training can blunt your *weight* loss, even as it increases fat loss. It will reduce inches, enhance body composition, change proportions, and boost energy. As a result, you can increase your expenditure of energy all day long. Depending on the circumstances, however, not lifting weights could make you lose weight faster. The issue is that more of your weight loss could be muscle when you're lifting weights. That's a formula for regain of at least the same as your loss, often more. That regain most definitely will be fat.

Choose your highest priority goal, and use the formulas in the next section to determine how much time and energy you want to spend on heavy, power, and light training. Of course, you want it all. You won't be completely ignoring the other benefits. You'll just optimize your approach to training to achieve the results that you want most.

❑ For Weight Loss

Heavy weight training results in a much higher post-exercise metabolism boost than lifting light weights. In fact, after performing heavy weight training, your metabolism can be anywhere from 15 percent to 75 percent higher hours after exercise, compared to using light weights. Such a result can have a major impact on how many calories you burn. Lift heavy and do it early in your workout, before you engage in functional training exercises. Focus on the major muscle groups. In that regard, the chest press, the row, and the leg press or squats are your major metabolism players.

Machine weights get a bad reputation from trainers, because they are stable and don't develop optimal balance and reaction skills. When you want to go heavy, however, stability is ideal. When you take away stability, you tend to forfeit the ability to lift heavy. As a result, therefore, you forfeit the most metabolism benefit. In this instance, machines can be your friends because they allow you to do heavy work safely. They have their place in your exercise routine.

A number of studies have found myth-busting results. For example, post-menopausal women who gained lean muscle following resistance training lost belly fat. The mistake you don't want to make when you're after belly fat loss is focusing on core exercises. At least not in the way that most people know "core." To a strength and conditioning coach, core exercise refers to squats, presses, and pulling exercises that engage your core for stability, while you use major muscles. The word and reference comes from core-of-the-workout exercise. You're not ever going to spot reduce in your belly, if you have all-over fat. Such a goal is a fairytale, Cinderella. Truth be known, lifting weights will result in a gain of overall lean muscle, as well as reduce belly fat faster than a Google search for the best ab exercises.

Power is your next best friend. After you have a foundation of strength and your joints and connective tissue have had several weeks, if not months, of training, change your routine by performing each repetition by lifting more rapidly and lowering more slowly to boost the energy expenditure of your workout. Keep in mind, however, that the hour you exercise is not sufficient to offset the 23 hours of inactivity you just endured. While some power is good, using heavy weight is still your first priority, if weight control and fat loss are your forever goals.

Lifting a light weight is optimal for enhancing gait and performing corrective exercises that strengthen those areas of your body in which you may have muscle imbalances. Such a regimen can help you move pain-free, as well as stay injury-free.

The ratio of time and energy you should devote to a heavy/moderate/light resistance level weight training workout is 50/30/20. Spend 50 percent of your time doing heavy weight, 30 percent using moderate weight to work on power, and 20 percent of your time performing light functional exercise. Plan each session and/or your total week with this kind of formula.

❏ For Bone Density

A routine that involves lifting heavy for 10 or fewer repetitions can have the most positive impact on your bones. If you want stronger bones, this workout is what you want to do. You may read about weight-bearing exercise (e.g., walking, jogging) and though they are better than non-weight-bearing exercise (e.g., biking, swimming), they only prevent further losses and only do that to a certain extent. They do not have what's referred to as a minimal effective stress (MES). In other words, your body is used to them, and you can do them repeatedly. They just don't have the impact on bones that you need for the most effect. The more time you spend in "unloaded" activities, like swimming, biking, or sitting, the more you need to load heavily in the weight room. Cardiovascular fitness, alone, does not have a direct correlation with your level of bone density.

Power also has positive effects on bone density. In fact, using heavy weight (which should be undertaken only after a good foundation of technique and adaptation have been established) with power has superior results to lifting weights slowly. Once again, the key is the amount of weight you lift. All factors considered, you can't achieve the bone density results you want/need by lifting light weight.

Not only does using light resistance benefit gait and balance challenges, it also can have a noteworthy impact on reducing fall risk. Ankle mobility and power, as well as (foot) plantar power and dorsiflexion, can improve by exercising on a regular basis with light resistance. In addition, such a workout can help reduce falls, strains, and sprains. The appropriate ratio of time and energy spent for bone density is heavy 40/power 40/light 20.

❑ For Sports Performance

Some of your exercise needs will be determined by your sport or leisure-time activity. For example, a shot put thrower has different exercise needs than a distance runner. Your workout routine will also be dictated, to a degree, by your goals to improve specific aspects of your performance. Injury prevention training will look different than efforts involving speed improvement, especially if you have an existing "niggle." For example, if you are an older runner who wants to improve your level of speed, you're going to spend less time in heavy lifting. Building up big muscles is not necessarily conducive to speed. On the other hand, you need some degree of strength to serve as your base for power.

Power movement, using moderate-to-heavy weight and performing fewer repetitions, is the area in which you want to spend the majority of your time. In this instance, a natural reduction in the number of repetitions your workout requires will occur, if for no other reason than when you're training for a sport, you should be spending time in the sport. As such, your focus should be on getting better at running, which means running more. For those older athletes who spend a lot of time in the pool or on a bike, this regimen also helps stave off bone losses.

Light resistance training is another good place to spend performance-enhancing time. Such an approach is often counterintuitive to an athlete who likes to "push" harder for better results. Oddly, injuries frequently result from the failure to do the "small" stuff, e.g., foam rolling (more on that topic in the rest and recovery chapter), ankle strength and mobility work, and one-legged work—all of which is low-resistance work. Doing hill training, with your own body weight, is a form of "light" resistance work. If you strength train the same day as hill work, you would leave out some of your leg work in order to not overtrain.

All factors considered, if you want to increase the level of function you achieve from your workout efforts, either when weight loss is not your primary goal or before it can legitimately be your main focus, you want to spend a significant amount of time performing light resistance training. Your heavy/moderate/light lifting ratio for enhancing sports performance and function, if your weight and body composition are not your major concerns, is 25/30/40.

No matter what your exercise goals are, you want to lift heavy, use power, and perform functional strength training with lighter weights. Managing the amount of time and the priority of each of these so that your workout regimen matches your goals and needs will help maximize your weight training efforts—emotionally, as well as performance-wise.

YOUR BIGGEST OBJECTIONS TO WEIGHT TRAINING

The elephant in the closet for women who don't strength train tends to be one of two things. Either you don't want to get hurt, or you don't want to get "bulky." These are notoriously the reasons why strength training has yet to become a habit for many women. If you're still thinking you'll try to get your sexy back without weight training and are a non-believer, read on. In reality, science shoots holes in both weight lifting fears.

Strength training programs targeted at improving lower body muscle power have been found to be well tolerated, safe, and effective, even among frail older adults (i.e., *really* older adults with high risk of falling). Medical and health/fitness professionals don't knowingly put subjects at undue risk. Ethically, they are not allowed to do so. As such, you are very likely stronger than the frailest elderly who have been studied.

Any fears you may have of gaining bulk will be hard for you to overcome. If you've previously experienced bulking up as a result of exercising, then it's natural you would assume it will happen again. Take a moment and reflect what else may have been going on at the time. Were you aware of proper work and recovery balance in your schedule? Many women who felt that they gained bulk by lifting weights subsequently realize that the diet they were following at the time contributed to their weight gain. Another possibility is that the protocol you used at the time wasn't right for your body type. In reality, there are hundreds of ways to manipulate sets, repetitions, and weight so that bulk doesn't happen.

Women don't have the right hormones to bulk easily. You've heard that before. For post-menopausal women, it's even more true. At age 50, not only do you have even less of the hormones that can bulk you up, you might be missing some of the fun you could be having by lifting weights.

Benefits from the weight room also extend to the bedroom. Traditionally, testosterone levels in women have not been a big focus of conversation. Until now, that is. When your libido drops, it can be a sign that your testosterone levels may also be lower than normal. One answer to that particular circumstance can be as easy as performing some quality weight training.

Besides feeling more confident in your body (clothed or naked), testosterone is your "alpha" hormone. It makes you a little bolder. Has your significant other ever objected to your intimate advances? It may just help in the boardroom too. Would your boss object if you took more initiative and spoke up? If you're the boss, would you like to be seen as a stronger leader? In other words, consider hitting the weights before the deli at noon.

SIZE DOESN'T DICTATE NEED

Sarcobesity is a term that describes being both fat and frail. As such, it is a double-bad aging cocktail for disease, falls, and isolation. Fear of falling, as well as an undue level of weakness, can keep you glued to your chair. The inactivity causes further weakening of muscles and an inability to react. You may not have the appearance of frailty, but you are not better and, in many cases, worse off than someone at a lower weight, if you fall. Strength training is one of the easiest ways to regain your confidence and the requisite level of function.

The right weight and repetition combination is mandatory for the results you want. Figure 4-1 summarizes how to select weight, according to your goals. Lifting speed is also important. Use a 1:1 or 1:4 ratio of lifting speeds, with 1:1 meaning lift slowly for four seconds and lower for four seconds. The 1:4 is done with a quick one-second lifting and a four-second lowering of the weight. If you're new to weight training or restarting after a time away from the weight room, use light weights and perform a few more repetitions than the end-goal repetition range. Start with 1:1, before you move on to power movements. Progress involves the neural component during that first six to eight weeks of working out such that a light weight does the job. In other words, train your brain first.

Weight	PCT	Repetitions	1:1 Ratio	1:4 Ratio	Benefits
Heavy	70-80%	<10-12	✔	✔	- Metabolism - Bone Density
Moderate	60%	=15	✔	✔	- Metabolism - Bone Density
Light	40%	<28		✔	- Gait - Power

Figure 4-1. The *After 50 Fitness Formula* weight lifting key

HOW FREQUENTLY SHOULD YOU TRAIN?

There are a variety of "right" answers to how often you should lift weights, which is part of the reason exercise can be confusing and may not get you results you need/want. The right number of days a week to train ranges from one to four times a week. There are different formulas for different people, based on different variables. How's that for an elusive answer? If you're left to figure it out yourself or to comply with someone else's schedule of sessions or classes, you might not have given much thought to it. You should.

In reality, a number of scientific studies on weight training have looked at the issue of frequency when working out. For example, one investigative research project, whose results appeared in the *Journal of Strength and Conditioning Research (JSCR)*, found that previously sedentary adults, i.e., individuals who spend an undue amount of time on the couch, derived the same results from lifting weights, regardless of whether they worked out one, two, or three times per week. On the other hand, with regard to the development of positive habits, exercise at a level of greater frequency, e.g., at least twice a week, might boost your level of stick-to-itiveness.

Physically, lifting one time a week can work for you, because during the first eight weeks of strength training, the changes you achieve are mostly the result of neuromuscular change. In other words, your brain is learning how to communicate with your muscles again. You start recruiting a few of the fibers to contract. Subsequently, your brain gets stronger, sending the signal to fire more fibers. After that initial period of six to eight weeks, you need a greater weight training frequency for optimal results.

In another study, whose results appeared in the *JSCR*, higher frequency led to better results in function for post-menopausal women who were *already exercising*. The subjects in this particular study strength trained three times a week. Keep in mind, however, that you have a real need for recovery. (Refer to the rest and recovery chapter for details.)

You also need to remember the importance of your psychological needs. In the previous example of working out once a week, such a regimen may not meet your habit-forming needs. In addition, you probably tend to like to keep a regular routine. Then again, easing into it one day a week may work for you. The key is to know yourself.

FAT CHANCE YOU'LL LOSE FAT IN EIGHT WEEKS

Body composition changes take time. There's a "get-it" factor for your brain. As you learn to recruit more muscles and focus on technique, you're laying a foundation. Most women want to go right to the penthouse and see the view. You want to see some fat loss from your labors. On the other hand, you should focus on the evidence that you're feeling stronger and feeling more confident. Shake that need for a scale or a body composition test to confirm that you feel better.

Your body is getting better at doing two things that will boost your ability to use, and therefore lose, fat. The fat has to be released so it's available to be used by muscles. Your ability to oxidize fatty acids also improves during the first few weeks of training. A program that includes cardio and resistance training will help you release and oxidize fat. When you start, it's as if you've been an overachiever in fat storage. Give your fat use and burning system a chance to catch up.

Another study found that adults over 60 who trained either two or three times a week achieved similar results. Researchers also found that heavy weight training has a threshold of no return. In other words, without adequate recovery between sessions, you can't see results. Not only does more make you tired, it doesn't necessarily get you better and might even get you worse results. This same study emphasized that while strength gains are obvious within eight weeks, body composition changes tend to lag behind. Significant improvements in lean body tissue and decreases in body fat tend to occur at 22 to 24 weeks. Be patient and stick with it. Keep in mind that you didn't achieve your current state overnight either.

You need to put science together with the collective art of your personality, life, and goals. Resistance training and cardio exercise both have many variables. The frequency, the exercises, and the number of sets and repetitions (which should dictate the weight you lift unless you're catering to an injured muscle or joint) all need to be taken into consideration. Once you've established your goals and know your own limits, you can establish the protocol that best meets your needs.

ESTABLISHING YOUR WEIGHT TRAINING SCHEDULE

If you like routine and have the time to exercise, you may want to lift three times a week. If you do, schedule it so that you have a minimum of 72 hours between your heavy days and add a lighter functional day in the middle. Functional exercises (e.g., those that focus on balance, gait, agility, and reaction) can be performed more frequently, since they require less recovery. For example, Monday lift heavy, Wednesday perform functional exercises, and Friday lift heavy.

If you choose two days a week due to time constraints or other reasons, its best to put those days 72 hours apart. On Monday and Thursday, for example, perform a complete session that includes heavy, power, and lighter weights. The more rest you have between workouts, the more lean muscle growth you'll get. Even if you've been lifting weights three days a week for years, you may find that increasing the amount of weight lifted and decreasing the frequency of your workouts to allow rest will reap more rewards for you. The harder you work during your sessions, the more rest you want between. You will get better results with less exercise, provided your training is focused and is at an adequate level of intensity.

HOW TO SELECT YOUR WEIGHT TRAINING EXERCISES

One of the biggest mistakes women make in the weight room is randomly using exercises. You need a plan. What and when you do what you do matters. Why it matters is fairly straightforward. For example, exercising your major muscle groups can have the greatest impact on your metabolism. What are your major muscle groups? Your chest, back, hip, and leg muscles are the major muscle groups in the body. Specifically, the major muscles are the pectorals, latissimus dorsi, trapezius, gluteals, quadriceps, and hamstrings.

Make no mistake, however, your smaller muscles are no less important to your whole-you fitness. Because they do not affect your metabolism in the same way, however, you need to discriminate. As such, the major muscle groups are the cool kids, and you need to spend more time with the cool kids, if you want to lose fat and keep lean.

The major muscles you want to focus on have one key factor in common—they cross more than one joint. When you do a pulling exercise, for example, both your shoulder and your elbow flex. When you perform a squat (sitting and standing qualifies), your hips and knees both flex and extend.

On occasion, your smaller muscles are the gatekeepers to metabolism-improving exercise. If you have a nagging shoulder injury or pain around an elbow, for instance, you may need to focus on your shoulder muscles initially in order to be able to safely lift with your larger muscles. You never want to ignore any muscles completely, whether you have an injury or not. You just need to prioritize what you do.

You can lift weights and still not be able to lift the water softener pellet bag out of the shopping cart into the car, let alone get it into your house and lift it to empty it into the water softener. Exercises that challenge you to carry heavy weights on one side or to use one leg or arm at a time are those most like your daily activities of life. If you enjoy sports, one-sided exercises can be very beneficial. Because you need a variety of resistance exercises, your next step should be to decide what ratio you need to lift—heavy versus light or machines versus balance challenges.

Tip: Use your smart phone and ear-phones while you lift weights. Watch a video describing the proper form, before you get on the machine. You'll get so much more out of the exercise. Find a trainer or a health/fitness club that provides this service.

DOES THE ORDER OF YOUR EXERCISE MATTER?

There are dozens of ways to sequence your exercises. The best way to sequence can be determined, in part, by how much time you have and what your priorities are. Recent studies have shown that sequence doesn't affect results as much as was once thought. It does matter which exercises you choose, however, if you have to make the most of 10 minutes. Exercising your shoulders or your biceps is not going to have the same effect on metabolism as using larger muscles.

It can also be very helpful for you to understand the full impact of how boot camps and cardiovascular interval training that incorporate weight training into your offerings fit into your strength training program. For example, programs that include high-intensity exercise, with relatively short rest periods, are designed to be very metabolically demanding. That feature may sound good, if you are aware that metabolically challenging means that you'll burn a lot of calories both during and after exercise.

When the exercise program includes both high intensity and short rest periods, however, the negative effects are also greater. For example, the amount of lactate and cortisol your body produces rises significantly, unless you're a well-trained athlete with a high level of fitness. Even coaches of well-trained athletes use caution with this type of training. If you're reading this book because you have hormones out of balance and can't seem to lose weight, sleep, or relax, the last thing you need is more cortisol.

This point is where your emotions can take over logic. You just want to work hard and get the weight off. You want more energy, and you want to stop feeling sick. You could easily think that performing more intense exercise, more often, and for longer is going to torch all those calories, and you will lose that fat in the process. Such a viewpoint couldn't be further from the truth.

Short-duration, high-intensity exercise one to two times a week, at most, with adequate rest, is the best formula to achieve increases in your hormone-healing metabolism. Overdoing high-intensity exercise, with too little rest, increases your level of cortisol, decreases the amount of growth hormone, and breaks down muscle. That combination leaves you tired, sore, and frustrated, while carrying the same amount of fat around.

You will also be at a greater risk of injury if you're not sleeping, have high stress levels, or are not eating adequate nutrients. This scenario is also a cocktail for adrenal fatigue. Remember that if you're doing things "right," and they aren't working, doing them more or harder is simply making matters worse.

Excess muscle damage from high-intensity exercise with a relatively short amount of rest is also possible. That's not your ticket to lean. You want lean muscle, *healthy* lean muscle, in order to fend off fat. Small doses of high-intensity exercise after a smart progression when the intensity level is slowly increased, makes sense only after your hormones are balanced. Beware of extreme exercise programs that are high intensity with relatively brief rest intervals or that are longer than 30 minutes in duration. They are sabotaging your hormone happiness.

If you perform resistance-training exercises in a class or a boot camp, consider that session as strength training. As such, you need to wait 48 hours before lifting again. This situation is one instance where many women neglect to see the whole picture accurately. For example, if you go to group-fitness classes and perform conditioning exercises with weights, each class counts as one weight training session. While it potentially isn't as effective as lifting heavier weight for developing fat free mass or bone density, you've still created fatigue and muscle damage. Whether you go into the weight room, or you use smaller weights at home or in a class, you have to rest between sessions when you exercise the same muscle groups. If you enjoy your group-fitness class and yet realize that you need some heavy lifting in your life, try doing an upper body push exercise, an upper body pull exercise, and a leg exercise with heavy weight, right after your class. Because it will only take no more than 10 minutes to do, you'll still be on track for rest and recovery.

HOW MUCH REST BETWEEN SETS OF EXERCISE?

The amount of time that you rest between sets of exercise deserves some consideration. Traditionally, when strength training, the heavier the weight and the more strength desired, the longer the interval of rest needed. At least two to three minutes of rest between sets has been found to provide optimal strength gains. In turn, a longer period of recovery was determined not to induce greater improvements.

While the amount of rest time doesn't seem to matter as much to younger trained athletes, even experienced resistance-trained older adults do better with more rest. In one particular study, young athletes, who rested two versus four minutes between sets, showed no difference in performance. Older adults did far better with more recovery between sets. All factors considered, the evidence indicates that yes, you can work as hard as you did when you were younger, as long as you rest more.

How do you fit the need for longer rest periods into your already all-too-brief time for exercising? If you perform a chest press, a row, and a squat in sequence, you could accomplish such an objective. Each exercise takes about a minute and a brief time to set up and move to the next exercise. By the time you return to the chest press a second time, you would have had adequate rest. You can plan a bigger circuit of major muscle group exercises, as long as you don't repeat a chest exercise with less than three minutes of rest. Lifting this way, you'll be optimizing your time and your results.

If you're doing more functional exercises, with light resistance, you don't need as much recovery. In fact, you could use a feeling of readiness as your gage. If you are performing sets of side-stepping with a band, rest briefly, and when you feel you can complete your next set with good form, begin again. If you find you can't get through the whole set, you learned you need a little longer rest period.

CAN'T YOU JUST DO CARDIO AND YOGA?

No! If you're still not convinced that you need strength training, this section is for you. Do you need cardio, strength training, *and* flexibility? Yes, you need them all. In studies comparing cardio only versus cardio and strength training combined, the most optimal results you can achieve come from the combined workout. On the other hand, if you have to choose between one or the other as you get older, you're going to find better results from strength training, than from cardio alone. You can't run from muscle or bone losses.

While yoga may seem like resistance training, and it is, it's not enough to help enhance your level of body composition, lean muscle tissue, or energy expenditure. If yoga helps you decrease stress-related cortisol, it absolutely will be a part of your weight loss efforts through hormone balancing. It's just not as beneficial as strength training will be on the muscular fitness bone density needs that should be the priority of every woman over 50.

Is it possible to lose the weight you've gained post-menopause? Yes. One study that looked at women, who were an average age of 63, who increased their level of both lean muscle and strength, as well as decreased their level of body mass and fat by performing resistance training twice a week, doing three sets of 6 to 14 repetitions per workout. That's just one study. In reality, there are dozens of examples out there, and many more underway. While it's going to take you finding muscle to lose the fat, you can absolutely do that … if you want to. The choice is yours.

Circuit training programs are one possible solution to reducing the time you exercise or the laundry you have to do. Within a single session of circuit training, you can move from exercise to exercise and include both strength and cardiovascular segments. Think of circuit training like a casserole. You mix up your strength and cardio exercises and move from one to the next, with a break for the muscles you just worked, while efficiently using time and keeping your heart rate elevated.

Studies have shown that circuit training elicits greater metabolic cost than treadmill training, when the two are matched for duration and energy expenditure. Both traditional strength training (with heavy weights) and circuit training give you higher post-exercise oxygen consumption than holding your same speed on the treadmill. The more oxygen you consume, the more calories you burn. Such a two-for-one option means that the energy you expend, while your body recovers after you exercise, makes the exercise that much more beneficial.

When circuit training, there is a metabolic boost with shorter rest periods and a strength boost with longer rest periods. Both approaches can help you spend more energy in the long run. It is possible to build a circuit that allows shorter rest between exercises and longer rest between exercises for the same muscle group. That scenario is the perfect formula for women after 50 who engage in weight training. The examples in Appendix B-8 should be used to get started. If you want the bottom line on the simplest way to boost your bottom line, the following guidelines should be applied:

- Lift twice a week.
- Put 72 hours between workouts whenever you can but never less than 48.
- Lift heavy early in your workout (fatigue at ≤ 10 repetitions).
- Perform compound exercises (e.g., squat, lunge, row, pulldown, chest press, etc.) first in your workout.
- Rest for three minutes between doing heavy sets for the same muscle group.
- Use power at least one day a week for each muscle group.

- Use light weight and one-sided exercises to improve gait and function.
- If you create a circuit, include enough exercises for approximately three minutes recovery between the same muscle groups.
- Eat protein before and/or after your resistance training exercise to optimize recovery and the benefit of your lean-creating exercise.
- Avoid doing the same routine every day you train. Vary the sequence, and the exercises, as well as the traditional routine versus circuit training, to keep your body guessing.
- Keep in mind that exercise is one of the only times in your day you want inefficiency. Muscle "disturbation" keeps you changing for the better.

While compound exercises that focus on two or major muscles at once are most beneficial for metabolism changes, you still want sexy arms right? There are ways to make those bicep curls and triceps extensions more effective. You don't have to ignore them. Just know that if you have limited time, working on your boomer booty will change your life more than working on your upper arms.

FEATURED EXPERT

Dan Ritchie and Cody Sipe

The Importance of Functional Strength (and How to Get It)

❑ What Is the Best Exercise After 50?

We ask this question when we speak to large groups, and the answer is almost unanimously "walking." Is walking really the best exercise for mature adults? It is easy to do, requires no special equipment or instruction, can be performed by almost anyone, and can be done pretty much anywhere at any time. It definitely has lots of advantages, but that doesn't make it the best. While cardiovascular fitness is an important component of function that we need to consider, it is only one piece of the puzzle.

❑ What About Strength Training?

"Stronger is better" is the mantra of today's fitness industry, but for the 50-plus adult, stronger is not always better. Do you really want massive biceps, ripped abs, and massive thighs … or have to spend hours in the gym every day in order to get them? Of course not. It's hard work. It doesn't feel good. And it doesn't give you the result that you *really* want … to be able to do the things you need to do, like to do, and want to do easier, better, and with less discomfort.

The science on this point is clear … being strong is important to be able to function, *but* once you are strong enough, then stronger isn't better. Think about it. How strong does your chest really need to be? How many activities in your day require a lot of chest strength? Well, unless you have a refrigerator fall on you, then probably not all that much.

Cardiovascular fitness and muscle strength are two components of functional fitness that need to be addressed, but there are many more that are equally, or even more, important, such as coordination, balance, mobility, joint flexibility, and core stability, to name a few.

❑ The Truth About Aging!

How well you age is up to you. The bad news is that after the age of 40, you are on a downward aging trajectory. Almost *all* of our physiological systems are in relative decline due to the aging process. The good news is that regular exercise and a healthy lifestyle can turn it around. *Most* of the bad stuff we attribute to aging is really due to a poor lifestyle, rather than the aging process itself. Fix the lifestyle, and essentially reverse or slow the aging process.

You don't think of yourself as a 50- or 60- or 70-year-old person, but you've noticed that your body can't quite keep up. You are a little heavier, a little slower, and a little weaker. Your knees don't feel so good, and you just don't have the energy you used to.

But, the good news is that you can get it all back with a functional strength training program designed with you in mind. The downfall of most traditional exercise programs for adults over 50 is that they are *way* too simplistic. They don't maximize functional results. They are designed for 20- to 30-year-olds and don't take the aging process into account. Furthermore, they are often painful or aggravating to perform. In reality, a functional strength training program can overcome all of these limitations, so that you regain and maintain a very high level of physical function for as long as possible.

As such, a functional strength program is distinctive in several ways:
- It gets you off weight-lifting machines and can be done with minimal equipment.
- It focuses on the integration of muscles working together, rather than on single-muscle strength.
- It provides lots of variety of movement patterns.
- It improves *all* of the essential elements of being able to move and live better.
- It addresses the distinct needs of someone in the second half of their life.
- It staves off boredom, because it is so much fun to do ("no pain, no gain"? I don't think so!).
- It can be performed much more quickly than traditional strength training programs.
- It uses light-to-moderate weights.

In just a matter of weeks, you will be climbing stairs with ease, getting down on the floor again to play with your grandchildren, traveling to exotic locations, spending hours in the garden, and doing all of the things you love to do, like you did 10 to 15 years ago! After all, isn't this what you *really* want out of a fitness program—to be able to live your life to the fullest for as long as possible?

Cody Sipe, PhD, is a professor, researcher, and award-winning fitness professional, who specializes in functional fitness for mature adults. He is co-author of the Amazon international best-seller Never Grow Old. For more information on functional strength training for mature adults go to www.functionalfitnesssolution.com.

Dan Ritchie, PhD, is a recognized authority on exercise and aging, an award-winning personal trainer, and vice president of the Functional Aging Institute. In his over 15-year career, he has helped thousands of adults over the age of 50, including those with chronic conditions, to regain their health, function, and quality of life through safe and effective exercise programs.

PART II: CARDIO EXERCISE

I'd proven to the world that maturity, experience, dedication, and ingenuity can make up for a little senescence. Muscle tightening is not the only thing that happens to our bodies over time. We gain knowledge, focus, and understanding, and those things can help us win.

—Dara Torres

Dara Torres said she was much more aware of what her body could do, as she returned to swimming as an older athlete. It empowered her, as long as she listened. She didn't work any less hard. She just needed more recovery. Diana Nyad, coincidentally also a swimmer, didn't dwell on the fact that she was *64*, swimming 110 miles from Havana to Key West. It was a feat for any age swimmer. Never underestimate the power of the human spirit is Nyad's message for us. Has your spirit grown or shrunk with age? When people ask you about your height, you say, "I used to be ____." Your spirit on the other hand has the ability to expand.

If you have begun to think that you can't do this or that because of the birthday that just passed, this chapter won't do you a lot of good. Decide before you read it whether or not you're willing to settle or not. If you defend your limitations, you get to keep them.

You may certainly have aches, pains, and prior or existing injuries. You may have a condition you have to work around. By age 50, many adults have at least one or two conditions. Some of them can be improved or reversed. More than 80 diseases can be prevented or treated with exercise. While you may have to work around pains and may have to choose your exercise type more carefully, you will feel better when you move. You are not as fragile as you might think.

WHAT SEPARATES YOU FROM YOUR YOUTH

Aside from joints and muscles that have a few more years of experiences on them, there are other things that can change the way you feel and age. Mitochondria are the "powerhouses of energy." If you get out of breath running upstairs or through the airport, you can blame it on your mitochondria. At least, you could have until now.

Not long ago, a natural decline of mitochondrial function was accepted as a part of aging. In the last 5 to 10 years, however, researchers have found otherwise. Both resistance training and endurance exercise can help turn mitochondrial function back 40 or more years within six months of training.

What does the aforementioned mean to you? It means more energy so that movement and activity are fun, rather than a chore. It means less unexplained breathlessness going upstairs. It can also help spare the effect of muscle loss caused by being inactive that increases your level of fat. The next factor will really make you want to bond with your mitochondria: it is your fat-burning furnace. You can increase your level of mitochondrial function with exercise. Motivated yet?

If a condition or joint pain restricts you, choose pain-free exercise and safety first. Then, focus on proper technique and instruction. Invest in a trainer. Use a video camera on your phone, if you need to, and record entire training sessions. Your investment in both the session and in the small inconvenience of creating a video can help you avoid setbacks, mistakes, or injury.

Putting firm muscle in the starring role and moving soft cellulite to the wings (not bat wings) requires both heavy breathing and pushing some weights around. Cardiovascular exercise, alone, won't do it. A study comparing runners who only ran with those who ran, as well as did strength training, found that you can't outrun muscle loss. In other words, you also can't out-Zumba, or out-elliptical, muscle loss.

Once you embrace weight training as a new best friend, you have to identify the type of strength you need. Refer to the strength section for specifics on resistance exercise. You can combine your cardio and your resistance exercise to reduce the time and frequency of exercise. First, define your goals and needs. If you want weight loss and bone density, you need to pull yourself off that cardio equipment and pump some heavier iron, even though your old habits may tell you otherwise. Exchanging even 10 minutes of cardio activity for concentrated strength training can improve your level of body composition and bone mineral density (BMD) most optimally.

Short bouts of high-intensity exercise and longer easy exercise for recovery will be your hormone healing pals. That's the focus of this section.

THE BURNING FAT QUESTION

The signs on the equipment that tell you the fat-burning zone involves a low heart rate are right. You're burning a high percentage of fat for fuel per minute. The problem is that your rate of overall calories burning is so low, that a high percent of a low burn is not much. The other misconception with heart rate charts is they'll give you a range, based on your age, that is simply not appropriate for most people. None of us fit that "average." If you work at a rate that is less than you need, you will achieve results that are less than you want.

When you exercise at higher intensities, you burn a lower percentage of body fat for fuel. The more fit you are, the more you're able to burn fat at a higher intensity. Even so, as Figure 4-2 illustrates, because you're burning calories faster, a low *percentage* of fat ends up being *more* fat. Dr. Len Kravitz, a University of New Mexico exercise physiologist, tested a subject working at two different levels of intensity. One intensity represented the so-called fat-burning zone, while the other was the equivalent of performing a high-intensity interval. The resulting level of total calories expended and the amount of fat calories used provides insight concerning the truth about fat-burning.

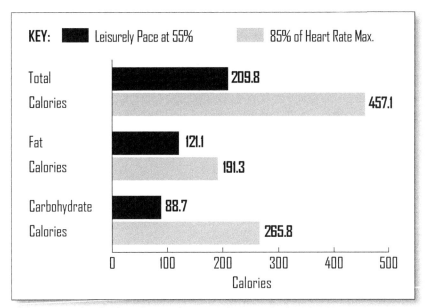

Figure 4-2. The fat-burning truth

Do you want to burn more fat *per minute* or more fat *total*, so it leaves your thighs alone? Treat that as a rhetorical question. The real excitement comes—hold onto your love handles—when you compare the amount of fat burned after different modes of exercise at different levels of intensities.

Scientifically, it's called excess post-oxygen consumption, or EPOC. Affectionately, you can call it passive fat loss. This "after-burn" is really what matters, when you're looking at the value of exercise for weight and energy management.

Resistance training—provided it's of sufficient intensity to overload your muscles—and cardio interval training have the highest after-burn. If you're thinking right now that intervals need to be your daily exercise, stop. On the other hand, if you just tuned out because you're an exercise-hater, I've got you covered too. Both doing intervals every day and never doing intervals will hurt your after-50 fat-loss fight.

There is a sweet spot for the right amount of exercise for you. Less than or beyond that point, more good doesn't happen, and more hormone imbalance can. The recovery chapter shares in-depth research on this factor. For now, know that in essence, too much exercise is just stress on your body. Stress causes cortisol. As noted previously, cortisol sabotages you with more cravings and less sleep. Too little sleep results in too little growth hormone, which you need to keep your sexy and curve-defining muscles.

Life is not measured by the number of breaths we take,
but by the moments that take our breath away.

—Maya Angelou

You need some moments that take your breath away. You need some high intensity exercise. A little of the right exercise will go a long way. If you're stressed and have weight gain, belly fat, and bat wings due to your hormones, the last thing your body needs is more stress.

If you go to an orthopedic surgeon with joint pain, the possibility of undergoing surgery is likely to come up. If you go to a physical therapist for joint pain, soft-tissue manipulation around the joint is probably going to come up. If you go to a chiropractor, spinal manipulation is probably going to come up. Not surprisingly, if you ask an interval instructor what's the best exercise approach for weight loss, intervals are going to come up. As a rule, we tend to follow the leaders who are already going in the direction we want to go.

You still need some of that long, slow exercise. Your inner cardio-queen just applauded. A dose-frequency adjustment is what you need. No one needs the "hour of power" every day. Maybe your inner cardio-queen was never born, and you're breathing a sigh of relief.

The most results-starved women are often suffering from experiencing the same level of intensity every day, or at least every day that they exercise. They pick random exercises classes, without thinking about the kind of exercise it is and how it fits their goals and needs. They have a flimsy plan for getting three days a week of exercise, as if it's optional. The biggest downfall of all is that they exercise without any intention. Having a purpose for each exercise session can help you get the results you want and expect. It takes consistent progressively challenging aerobic exercise, sprinkled with recovery days, to develop your body as a "fat burner."

For results that help you look good and feel great, your exercise choices matter. Random exercise gets random results. The recent trend in high intensity interval training (HIIT) favors both shorter workouts and more optimal fat utilization from the burning of calories that occurs after (not during) the exercise. Those are two seductive reasons you could easily fall in love with and think intervals are the way, the only way, to exercise. Intervals are a part of a complete exercise program after 50, but not the only part.

INTERVAL ANSWERS

How do intervals work and how do you use them optimally for you and your hormone balance? The following five points can help address these issues:

❑ #1. More Is Not Better

One to three times a week is the most you want to do intervals. The woman's way is often if a little is good, more is better. For the over-50 crowd, recovery is key. You can work hard, just as hard as when you were younger, but you will need more recovery between performing your intervals. A week may become a nine-day cycle of exercise, similar the sample in Figure 4-3. It might not make sense for you to do Monday-Wednesday-Friday classes anymore. If you've been exercising too frequently, you might be pleasantly surprised to find your level of fitness (e.g., energy, ability to sleep, fat loss, etc.) improves with two days of rest between intense exercise sessions.

	DAY 1	DAY 2	DAY 3	DAY 4	DAY 5	DAY 6	DAY 7	DAY 8	DAY 9
	High-Intensity Intervals Heavy Weight Training	Recovery -Yoga -Stretch -Pilates	Long Slow Day	Heavy Weights & Balance Training High-Intensity Intervals	Recovery -Yoga -Stretch -Pilates	Long Slow Day	Mid-Length Intervals Heavy Weight Training	Long Slow Day	Rest Day

Figure 4-3. Sample nine-day exercise plan

Start your interval training wisely, with one session a week. It's easy to do the opposite. You get pulled into a class that is offered at specific days and times, and you register. You're trying to fit your fitness level, status, and needs into an existing blueprint. Break the mold! You don't get your money's worth by going more days of the week, but by getting more fit. The results are what matters. Anyone can get tired. You want to get fit. You still want to be active, just at a variety of intensity levels. Exercise classes built for routine and the masses may not fit your need for recovery. You simply need more time between sets and between sessions. Start asking about something that fits you better. For optimal results, sans being injured, adhere to the following guidelines concerning how frequently you should engage in interval training:
- If you're a newbie to intervals: one day a week
- If you're already doing intervals: one or two days a week, with 72 hours between. If it's a must for your schedule, 48 hours is OK, but not ideal.

- If you've already been doing intervals consistently for six months: one to three days a week, but experiment with rest. Three days of intervals in a nine-day cycle may work best.

You live and breathe by a seven-day week. While it may be tempting to try to fit your exercise needs into the seven-day schedule, your results and level of motivation may be better, if you use a nine-day exercise plan. It could be worth doing a three- or four-week trial.

❑ #2. Use the 80/20 Rule

Whether you want to get faster, fitter, or firmer, the 80/20 rule applies to the amount of time you spend doing intervals. Only 20 percent of your time should be interval time. More really isn't better. The other 80 percent should focus on the foundation of your level of cardiovascular fitness. Life, after all, is about stamina and endurance. We have to sprint sometimes, but more sprinting doesn't make you fitter faster. You still want long walks. You still want some moderate-duration, moderate-intensity exercise. Sprinkle intervals into your training routine, rather than focus only on them. Plan your exercise sessions this way, and your exercise will become more effective.

For example, say you do (not a suggestion yet!) a 30 x 30 x 30 interval workout. That's 30 seconds of "hard" and 30 seconds of recovery done 30 times. The total interval time = 15 minutes. At this point, look at your total amount of time spent exercising. You have 30 minutes of interval/recovery time, and with a 10-minute warm-up and cool-down each, you'd have a total of 10 + 30 + 10 = 50 minutes. The "work" intervals take 15 minutes and the remainder of the workout is 35 minutes. In other words, you've devoted 33 percent of your total workout time to intervals in this example.

If your week includes two long (40 minutes each) walks (a total of 80 minutes) and one other day of performing 10 minutes of hard interval time during a short 20-minute workout, in addition to the aforementioned 50-minute session, your exercise routine would have 25 total minutes of intervals and 125 minutes of "other" exercise time for the week. In other words, 20 percent of your exercise efforts for the week involved doing intervals. Such a smart approach to exercising (one that includes recovery exercise) will increase your level of both fitness and energy, instead of breaking you down over and over again.

You don't have to sit down and do the math constantly, but an occasional snapshot can be worth the time. When you wonder why you're not seeing results, or you're exercising but are tired, this hypothetical scenario could shed some light on the reason.

❑ #3. Work Time ≤ Recovery Time When You're Beginning

A sound fitness regimen always involves a progression. While the goddess in your head that is engraining in your mind an idea of what a bathing suit fitting should look like and that in order to achieve such an ideal, you want more results faster, adopting such an attitude will leave you frustrated with an enhanced likelihood of being injured, but not necessarily fit. If you undertake the aforementioned 30 x 30 x 30 workout for example, which involves a 1:1 ratio of work to recovery, you might be OK with doing that. If you're just beginning to do intervals, however, a better approach might be to reduce the number of intervals from 30 to 15, and employ a 30-seconds work:60-seconds recovery regimen.

You want to be able to recover. In other words, you want to be breathing easier at the end of your recovery time. Over weeks of training, you will recover faster. Don't allow your intervals to get "cloudy," i.e., when your form deteriorates and you're not able to do as much work during work and your ability to recover isn't really recovered. Clearly, work hard, and recover easy. Sometimes, in order to manage such an approach, you might have to "skip" an interval and start again with the next interval.

❑ #4. How to Interval

Speed or resistance can both work as intervals. Walking up a hill outdoors, without losing speed, is resistance. Research suggests that the risk of being injured is slightly greater with speed, than with resistance. You can do your intervals in the pool, outdoors, or using equipment.

You might mistakenly think high-impact exercises, like running or jumping, have to be involved. Not so. Anything can work. Performing squats with body weight or with added resistance from a weighted vest or dumbbells can be your interval. Boxing is an example of a fun way to get cardio intervals. Biking faster or with more resistance is intervals. Just about anything you name can become interval training. Even with a small space to exercise, you have options. In fact, you may realize that you have been doing some form of interval training already.

❑ #5. Length of Intervals

Typically, shorter intervals work a different system than longer intervals. Start with short ones, 30 seconds in duration. You want them to be "doable" and to provide you with a feeling of success. It doesn't take much to see real progress and feel entirely different after exercising. Longer intervals, of at least two minutes in duration, seem to have a greater impact on your overall level of fitness. They elevate what's called your $\dot{V}O_2$max. As a result, you can do more—during life as well as exercise—without getting fatigued. This increase in interval length should be of interest to you if you would like to develop more stamina and endurance.

If you're looking for weight management and a way to exercise in a relatively short amount of time, you might decide to stick with short intervals on your interval days. Don't attempt a two-minute interval right out of the interval gate. Build up over weeks and even months. Furthermore, don't attempt four sets of short intervals back-to-back right away. More is not just more. More is often too much. When you get tired, you lose form. In turn, you'll have a greater risk of being injured. Refer to the chapter on recovery for *more* on that.

SAMPLE INTERVAL WORKOUTS

The following simple interval workouts illustrate two examples of how you could structure your interval training. One workout is for you if you're a beginner, and one is for you if you already have been doing intervals.

❏ Beginner's Interval Workout

- Warm up for 10 minutes.
- Perform :30 work to 1:00 recovery x 10.
- Cool down at least five minutes.

❏ More Experienced Exerciser Interval Workout

- Warm up for 10 minutes.
- Perform :30 work to :30 recovery x 30.
- Cool down at least five minutes.
- Add to or exchange this workout for one of your exercise days.

Life has natural intervals. At every age, intervals are a beneficial part of exercise. While special conditions might challenge you or your trainer, they don't have to prevent you from doing interval training. For example, emphysema patients do intervals. In fact, they do better with them than longer steady exercise.

THE SEE-HOW-I-FEEL WORKOUT

Too often, individuals have no plan. They have a vague intention to exercise, but haven't really put it on their calendar. Worse, they have no idea of what the workout goal is and what they're going to do to accomplish it.

There are two problems with this situation. One is if you're like a lot of women, you feel stressed, rushed, and crushed for time. In those circumstances, exercise is usually the first to go from your schedule. At the end of the day, it's too easy to feel like wine and dine, instead of weights and cardio. At the other end of the spectrum are the amazing workouts that feel like you can do anything and everything. Unfortunately, all too often, they can result in an injury.

"I felt so great, I just kept going." No, no, no. You *should* feel good. Go right ahead and feel good. Just stop, when you planned to stop.

FLEXIBILITY IS THE PLAN

Life can be messy. You'll have interruptions, hiccups, and mornings when you wake scheduled for a big workout not feeling well or didn't need to wake up because you were up! Adjust to the circumstances. Whether it's missing a workout or cutting the duration and intensity of your workout in half, responding is smart. If you're a type A person, disciplined and think gutting out a tough workout is virtuous, think again. You're already on a hormone roller coaster if you're sleep-deprived, for instance. You slow your progress when you ignore the need to respond to things that life throws at you.

Resist the desire to "make it up" if you miss. Don't double the workout the next day. Whether or not exercise stress plays a part in you not feeling 100 percent this time, it most likely will in the future, if you try to play "catch up."

The more wisely you plan your exercise schedule, the less illness and poor sleep will plague you. Exercise boosts your immune system and improves the quality of your sleep, when you take it in the right dose. There are a dozen right ways to plan an exercise schedule. There are probably fewer for you, when you factor in the rest of your life, the time of day you want to or need to exercise, and the activities you like. Previously, a nine-day exercise plan was detailed that allows for more rest and recovery. Because the rest of your life is based on a seven-day week, you may find it's easier to plan your exercise that way. Figure 4-4 details a plan that includes some flexibility (not to be confused with yoga). Notice that rest and recovery days follow or precede more challenging days. If you're just starting out and habit, not intensity, is your first goal, this seven-day plan may suit you well.

Monday	Tuesday	Wednesday	Thursday	Friday	Saturday	Sunday
Short Intervals	Rest Day	Longer Intervals	Recovery Day	Heavy Weights	Rest Day	Long Slow
Heavy Weights		Functional Weights	Yoga			

Figure 4-4. Sample *After 50 Fitness Formula* weekly plan

THE BEST TIME OF DAY TO EXERCISE

If you're smiling, it's potentially because you think you know the answer to this age-old question. The best time of day to exercise is the time you will actually exercise! That's always been the health/fitness professional's answer. Then, there's the reality that first thing in the morning is the least likely time to be interrupted and the most likely time to set you up for making good health choices all day.

You may have a well-established schedule for exercise. On the other hand, your hormones may have a different idea of what constitutes an optimal schedule for you. Stress, lack of sleep, and afternoon cravings suggest high cortisol levels. Work with, rather than against, your hormones by doing more vigorous exercising in the morning. Your (short) interval training, strength training, or combination thereof will optimize your cortisol use when it's at its highest—in the morning. Late in the day, include taking an easy walk outdoors or doing yoga, activities that help reduce your level of cortisol and prepare you for sleeping. Keep in mind that if you're yoga-phobic for some reason, yoga won't be at all stress reducing. The point is, use activities that are lower intensity and relaxing for *you*.

If the time of day you exercise is dictated by how you pay the bills, do the best you can to create a hormone-happy schedule. It may be helpful for you to take advantage of your weekends and insert rest days into your week in order to have more control over the scheduling of your exercise efforts.

You can monitor your intensity level in a number of ways. Figure 4-5 represents both subjective and objective measures. The following paragraphs detail your options and how they are related to each other.

Zone	% Max HR	RPE (1-10)	Type of Exercise	Breath	Talk	Duration	Frequency
1	50-60%	2-3	Recovery	Nose	Normal talk	15 minutes to several hours	1-3 times a week
2	60-70%	4-5	Endurance	Nose	Mostly complete sentences	≤75 minutes	1-3 times a week
3	70-80%	6-7	Tempo	Nose-mouth	Between breaths	15-35 minutes	1-2 times a week
4	80-90%	8-9	High-intensity intervals	Mouth	Choppy, one word	10-40 minutes in intervals	1-3 times a week
5	90-100%	9-10	All-out sprint	Heavy mouth	Hand gestures	≤1 minute at a finish line	1-3 times a week

Figure 4-5. The *After 50 Fitness Formula* intensity chart

The percentages included in Figure 4-5 are related to your maximum known heart rate. Standardized formulas have proven very unreliable, especially for adults over 40. The best way to really know is to have them tested. If you calculate your heart rate, based on a formula, or use a chart on the wall, based on your age there's a strong chance it will either over- or underestimate what you should do. If you exercise at a heart rate range too low, you may not be affecting your fitness level. On the other hand, exercising harder than you should can result in a hormone imbalance from overtraining. You can also get along just fine without ever testing your heart rate. Even if you're taking medications that blunt or increase heart rate, the subjective measures listed in Figure 4-5 will work just fine for you.

The rating of perceived exertion (RPE) scale is based on a 6-20 rating by Victor Borg. A modified 1-10 scale is more user-friendly. Using this "how-you-feel" rating will help you connect to more objective evaluations of your exercise. If you also monitor heart rate, you may see a pattern or an anomaly. If you're tracking distance covered in a specific time, in combination with RPE, you will see proof that you're becoming more fit, as you cover more ground with the same or lower RPE. There's more on this 1-10 scale later in this chapter.

The type of exercise describes the variety of exercise you want to include in each week for optimal fitness. Start with a foundation of low-zone work to build an anaerobic base. Next, add interval training and some longer, but lighter, recovery days. A well-rounded fitness program features one of each every week and might repeat one or more types, depending on your goals, as well as your schedule, on occasion. Recovery days can include activities, such as hiking or golfing that can last a long time but are at relatively low intensity levels. You can also do light and short versions of your harder activity days. Low-impact activity is best. A few laps (swimming or walking) in the pool or a 30-minute light spin (on a cycle) can serve as a recovery day. Don't be tempted to go longer such that your exercise efforts become a workout.

The breath-and-talk test will help you decide if you're in the right zone for your exercise-session goal. If you're doing a recovery day, and you can't talk, you need to reduce the speed or resistance level at which you're doing training. On the other hand, if you're doing an interval, and you can still talk in complete sentences, it's time to dial it up sister!

Duration and frequency on the heart rate chart are only broad ranges. They'll vary, based on your level of fitness and any time constraints you may face. If you're just starting or restarting and/or are highly stressed, choose the lower frequency and least amount of time. This is the point at which you need to pay attention. The activity you *like* is probably not the one you need to do more. Huh? Yes, you're busted. If you love long, slow walking, what you really need is interval training to balance your weekly routine. Don't think you're progressing by just adding more of what you're already doing.

The amount of time you spend in each zone is illustrated in Figure 4-6. The amounts may surprise you. Zone 1 represents a strong foundation of daily activity sprinkled through your waking hours. Non-exercise activity time (NEAT) is critical to your overall efforts at metabolism-boosting, as well as joint and muscle care. It's been well-established that an hour of exercise three times a week does not make up for 23 hours a day being sedentary. Zone 2 is easy, slow, longer endurance and again a big part of your fitness base-building. Don't get seduced by high intensity interval training so much that you dump your relationship altogether with long and slow. It's OK to play the field. Flirt with all of them.

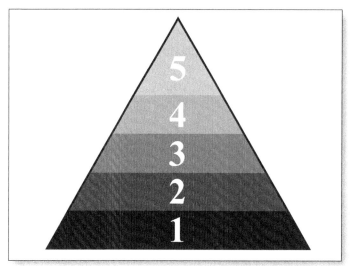

Figure 4-6. Cardiovascular training zones

Cardio intervals usually range from 30 seconds to three minutes. If you happen to be training or have for a longer event, like a 5K or a triathlon, you have experienced longer intervals of working in higher zones. This chapter focuses on mostly shorter intervals for fitness and fitness base-building. Optimal-hormone balancing exercise, if you want to lose weight but can't, or are exercising, but find you have no energy, involves training of shorter duration. Your *After 50 Fitness Formula* looks different than either your 30-something formula or a class for the masses does.

How do you know if you need to change your approach? If you notice you're going along fine and your progress slows, it's time for a change. If you notice you're suddenly suffering more injuries and more niggles, it's not just "getting older." You're either not recovering according to your body's current needs, or you're not exercising consistently enough. You haven't found your "Goldilocks" exercise routine. There are plenty of uninjured older athletes and fitness enthusiasts.

TABATA

The queen of the interval-training tabloid is Tabata. Tabata features 20 seconds of high-intensity intervals, followed by 10-second bouts of recovery, sequentially done eight times in a four-minute set. Express classes (i.e., a condensed express session that typically is scheduled for 30 to 45 minutes or less) suggest that you rest a minute and then begin again, getting up to four sets of this intense work in 20 minutes. It's quite advanced and based on research with elite cyclists. In the original study, the cyclists were used to challenging workouts and performed work intervals at 110 percent of their max. You can interpret that scenario as uncomfortable.

This protocol is not ideal for a beginner boomer babe. It may also be too much, even if you're more experienced, but have high levels of stress and cortisol. Twenty minutes sounds attractive though and anyone desperate for fat-burning benefits could fall for it. By the time you do all-out sprints for even 20 seconds eight times, however, your form is going to fall apart. That's where risk of injury creeps in and separates you from your vision of svelte, sexy boomer babe.

The smart starting point for doing intervals is to have a recovery period that is equal or longer to the work level. For instance, you could perform a 30-second interval, with a 30- or 60-second recovery. You could even recover for 90 seconds or for 4:30. Another example of a possible interval workout would be to perform a steady workout, but with a 30-second burst at the end of each five-minute set. Such a workout would provide you with both a mental break and a chance to work your fast-twitch fibers, as well as your reaction skills.

The sidebar on the next page shows a sample featuring longer intervals. The workout itself is moderate in length. There are five intervals that suggest different options. You'll see how you can combine cardio and resistance training within a session or keep it all more cardiovascular.

If you try to maintain the same speed throughout your workout, you may notice that either your level of exertion or your heart rate (or both) creeps up. Adjust your intensity level, based on how you feel, not on what speed the machine says. You want to keep that zone 2 feeling of a "5" on a 1-10 scale, without allowing yourself to get so fatigued you lose form.

To progress, you can play with several variables. Change one at a time for best results. If you focus on total volume of time in work intervals, you're calculating what matters:

- 8 x 20 seconds with 10-second recovery = 2 minutes and 40 seconds
- 30 x 30 seconds with 30-second recovery = 15 minutes
- 5 x 3:00 with 3 minutes rest = 15 minutes

Notice that the work-interval duration multiplied by the number of times the work interval is repeated gives you the total work volume. The recovery time can be according to your status as just starting out or more experienced. As you increase your level of fitness, you will recover better. Naturally, over the course of a workout, your heart rate will rise easier and your recovery will take longer. Your first couple of intervals will feel fine, and your last couple will also feel *fine*.

How do you challenge yourself progressively? You can increase the number of intervals you perform, if you have the time. You can also increase the duration of the intervals (and the length of the recovery). Furthermore, you could decrease the time of the recovery. For example, from 30-second intervals and a 60-second recovery, you could progress to 30-second intervals, with a 30-second recovery. Then, you could do 60-second intervals and a 60-second recovery. Eventually, you could do 60-second intervals and a 45-second recovery. To check whether or not you've made a drastic leap or a reasonable one, sit down and do the math on the total time in work and recovery intervals.

❑ *Warm up progressively by increasing the intensity level by either increasing the speed of the exercise or doing additional resistance in the chosen cardio activity for five minutes*

❑ *Walk/bike/swim/dance for 4:30, progressively getting faster (zone 2: 5 RPE)*

❑ *30-second "sprint" or perform a body weight goblet squat (zone 3-4: 9 RPE)*

❑ *Repeat cardio for 4:30 at an RPE exertion level of 5 on a 1-10 scale (zone 2)*

❑ *30-second "sprint" or do alternating rear lunges (zone 3-4)*

❑ *Repeat cardio for 4:30 at an RPE exertion level of 5 on a 1-10 scale*

❑ *30-second "sprint" or do alternating side lunges*

❑ *Repeat cardio for 4:30 at an RPE exertion level of 5 on a 1-10 scale*

❑ *30-second "sprint" or do a push-up (you can use the wall)*

❑ *Repeat cardio for 4:30 at an RPE exertion level of 5 on a 1-10 scale*

❑ *30-second "sprint" or do a renegade row (a plank with a weighted row)*

❑ *Cool down with three to five minutes of walking*

Mix longer and shorter intervals on different days of the week to increase your level of fitness endurance and boost your $\dot{V}O_2$max. For example, you could do short 20- or 30-second intervals on Monday, and then use Friday to perform increasingly longer intervals, building up to three minutes over many weeks.

Your intervals can be done with either all cardio, a combination of cardio and strength training, or primarily strength training, all with a proper warm-up. If you're using strength training, you'll want to focus on the major muscle groups and compound exercises to help elevate your heart rate to achieve the desired training effect.

Squats, lunges, push-ups, and bent-over rows are compound exercises. Leg extensions and bicep curls are not. A hamstring curl, using a ball, qualifies as a compound exercise. Compound exercises simultaneously incorporate multiple muscles and joints.

Why are intervals so popular? Oxygen consumption is related to calorie burning. If you boost your level of fitness, you will naturally burn more calories all of the time. In other words, you boost your level of metabolism more than by simply doing steady, slow exercise on an ongoing basis.

When you perform intervals, the underlying objective is to get breathless. You want to have earned the recovery interval. If you're just increasing a speed on the bike or treadmill to another comfortable level, and then decreasing for the assigned recovery period, you won't see the results you want, including a boost in fat-burning post-exercise.

No one can tell you, without first testing you, at what speed to exercise on a treadmill. Even if they could, it will change as your level of fitness increases. In a similar vein, no one can tell you what heart rate to shoot for in a short interval, because a heart-rate monitor can't keep up. Even a coach who tests you can't always predict how you will respond on a given day or how quickly or slowly you'll adapt. That's good news, because it means that the answer to your quest lies in you.

Using a rating of perceived exertion (RPE) scale enables you to know how you feel. How you feel doesn't lie. When you do short interval bursts of 30 seconds, a heart-rate monitor really can't keep up. It doesn't reflect an accurate heart rate for the interval. While a heart-rate monitor can be better used for longer intervals, it isn't required. Even if you use a heart-rate monitor, a combination of heart-rate monitoring and your own RPE is ideal. As such, you'll have both an objective and a subjective measure. The following 1-10 scale guide is an example of a personalized RPE:

- #1—lying on the couch
- #2—sitting up on the couch, using the remote control
- #3 and #4—daily activities of life, e.g., flying up and down the stairs to do laundry; whirling through the grocery store; raking the lawn; etc.
- #5—steady exercise, at an intensity level that you could maintain for an extended length of time
- #6—activity at a slightly higher, but still comfortable, level
- #7 and #8—the activity, e.g., longer intervals, gets more interesting and you're beginning to watch the clock
- #9—shorter intervals, eventually becoming an all-out sprint
- #10—activity, such as running to a finish line, which takes only a few seconds; all factors considered, you don't purposely undertake this activity or spend much time doing it

An example of a newbie interval workout is doing 30-second intervals, aiming for an RPE rate of "9" and recovery intervals that take you back down to an RPE rate of "2 or 3." If you're on an exercise bike, you can choose a baseline cadence of 90 revolutions per minute (RPM), and then add either speed or resistance during the interval. The 85 to 100 RPMs is the optimal power range. If you can't reach that speed yet, use your highest comfortable RPM as your set pace. To increase the level of intensity, add resistance.

If you want to increase your level of fitness and energy, and keep your weight under control with a crazy schedule doing short intervals, one to three (once your hormones are in balance) days of the week is a good plan to achieve your goals. Always start with the least level of frequency for at least a few weeks. You have to find your sweet spot. An all-intervals-all-the-time approach is neither good for your hormones nor a good fitness strategy. Complement your interval training with a long session of performing your favorite activity at least once a week, as well as engaging in a moderate day or two. All signs should point to feeling better. Exhaustion and poor sleep are signs that you still need to tweak your workout for the right fit.

AVOID TOO MUCH OF A GOOD THING

If you're that woman who exercises at the same intensity, same duration, doing the same dreadmill or elliptical workout every day, beware. You've seen her. She's at the gym every day, but her body never changes. She exercises twice as much as most individuals do, but she looks the same. Even worse, she may, in fact, be heavier, have more fat, or have a tight, drawn face.

There is a threshold of no returns. In other words, you slave away at exercise—of any type—and, at some point, you just don't get a return for your efforts. As research has shown, it's clear that more exercise actually prevents you from getting the return you deserve. Less exercise can be more when it comes to results. Less volume and the right exercise are the most beneficial for hormone balancing. Weight loss and energy gains occur easier and more naturally when you find your Goldilocks spot.

Too much cardio can spike muscle-eating stress hormones, like cortisol, as well as hinder thyroid hormones, leading to fatigue and *slowed* metabolic rate (the rate at which you burn calories at rest). That's a formula for losing belly fat. You simply can't get fit, while you're exhausted. Plus, too-frequent long, moderate-intensity aerobic workouts tend to reduce your levels of the satiating hormone leptin, making you ravenous afterward. In contrast, the optimal frequency of short, intense cardio sessions (in addition to strength training) stimulates fat-burning hormones like testosterone and human growth hormone to boost metabolism.

If you're short on exercise time, try 30- to 45-minute workouts, one or two times weekly, combining intervals (cardio bursts punctuated by brief periods of rest) and strength training. On your "off" days, walk for 30 to 60 minutes. If you're just starting out, begin with one interval day per week for two weeks. When you add a second day, vary either the mode of aerobic activity or the strength training exercises you do.

Studies show that more exercise (than you need) can lead to less activity all day long. Non-exercise activity thermogenesis (NEAT) can have a positive impact on your best boomer body. If you overwork yourself in the gym and sit the rest of the day, as occurred with the participants in the study who did more exercise than they needed, your overall energy expenditure, over the course of a day, will go down. As such, you will couch-compensate. In the latter study referenced, older female subjects, who exercised formally just twice a week, had greater level of weekly energy expenditure than those who worked out three or more times per week. Not only did they boost their level of energy, they were also more inclined to want to golf, hike, garden, or tackle their house-cleaning chores.

WHAT ABOUT BONES?

Bone mineral density (BMD) is most optimally affected by a combination of dynamic weight-bearing exercise and heavy-load resistance training. You can read more about resistance training for BMD in the strength training section of this chapter. How much does weight-bearing cardio help bone density? All factors considered, it has a minimal impact. After 50, because you're less inclined to do a lot of jumping, leaping, and landing with high impact, your cardiovascular exercise tends to contribute less to your total bone density.

The best combination that has been documented for bone density is doing weight-bearing exercises, like jogging, jumping, and vibration, paired with heavy weight training. If you have access to a vibration machine, several studies have found that its use can generate bone density improvements at the hip with it. On the other hand, if you are apparently healthy and can lift heavy weight, you can do as much good in 10 minutes of quality weight work as you can with a vibration machine.

If you are sedentary and begin a jogging or jump-rope program, you'll experience a boost in bone density, compared to a lifestyle spent on the couch. If you've been jogging for years, however, you're not gaining more bone-density benefits, though you may be helping to maintain your level of bone density, at least in your lower body. If you are a runner who begins to swim and bike more, you will incur less bone-density benefit from those cardio options, since they are not weight-bearing. On the other hand, that's not to say they aren't wonderful modes of cardio exercise that can help provide you with excellent balance in your overall level of fitness, as well as help prevent overuse of your musculature. They just don't help you meet the minimal effective stress (MES) required to gain stronger bones. As such, the repetitive nature of walking or jogging is not as effective as doing a few heavy load repetitions.

Performing dance and mind-body exercises (e.g., Zumba or yoga) might, however, make you less prone to falling because you have better balance and reaction skills. While the aforementioned doesn't directly help prevent low bone density or osteoporosis, it is a viable way to prevent fractures from falls.

BEFORE YOU BEGIN: CHECK YOUR READINESS

If you have not been training regularly, the following questions should be answered before you begin:

- Do you have heart problems, high blood pressure, bone, or joint problems that could be worsened by exercise?
- Do you frequently suffer from chest pains, feel faint, or have dizzy spells?
- Are you taking any prescription medications?
- Is there another medical reason why you should not exercise? (Never forget that most likely, there are plenty why you should!)

If you answered "yes" to any of the aforementioned questions, consult your physician before beginning your training program. Then, do it. There are far more reasons why you should, than why you shouldn't, exercise.

Kymberly Williams-Evans, MA, and Alexandra Williams, MA

❑ Cardio for Boom-Chicka Boomers: Walk (or Run?) to the "Best" Cardio Workout

As longtime fitness leaders, we are often asked, *"What is the best cardio workout?"* The bottom line is that the "best" activity is the one you will actually do. Log the time and intensity level of your exercise efforts. Which activity do you find most comfortable on your body? Which one will you stick with the longest? Which one keeps you injury free? Your goal should be to go as long as you can, as hard as you can, as often as you can. What do you actually *like* doing? Yes, it's that simple and accessible!

The exact "right" one depends on you. Do you prefer cardio machines, group classes, or outdoor activities? Are you a walker or a runner? You have to do the one that you will actually do! What? That sounds like a skanky date proposal!

Even better, is to change up the activity or select several enjoyable aerobic modes. You might do a step class one day, walk the next, take a swim later in the week, and then top off the weekend with a session on an elliptical machine. (Moseying through the mall does not count, even if your heart rate elevates at the good deals!) If you always power walk, try a stair-climber now and then. If you always run on a treadmill, join a fitness class that gets your heart rate up.

We could give you heart rate formulas and a discussion about involved joints and high-impact versus medium or low-impact, but why get caught up in all that? "Log your time; be happy" is the best advice we can give you for cardio. Your body will tell you what you prefer doing. "Log time," by the way, refers to writing down the amount of time you are doing your chosen activity. You don't get to count the time spent "standing in the shade" or "checking phone messages." Walking is one of our favorite non-work-related aerobic exercises, because it allows us ample time to play with our camera phones. We can't take great shots if we're running!

❑ Cardio Is Dead: Long Live Cardio

Now that you have tossed aside the constraints of "this is better than that," and embraced the happy place of choosing activities you enjoy, you might have landed on the second most popular cardio question: "how much aerobic exercise do I need?"

Have you seen recent headlines telling us to "forget cardio exercise. since it's a waste of time," followed by "perform aerobic activity nearly every day!" Mamma mia. What are we to do if we want to get more fit? Are you confuzzled yet? Just recently, we read an article entitled: "Newsflash: Cardio Is Dead." As longtime fitness pros and proponents of aerobic exercise, we were bothered by this announcement in a cranky, "oh, great, now people will exercise even less" kind of way.

Is cardio really "dead?" Or, are we going to be soon, if we stop doing aerobic exercise and drop even more activity from our lives? For years, we've been told to work out aerobically five to six days per week. Now, we're told to forego it. What fitness tips should we follow and what hype can we safely ignore? *How can you know what actions to take* (aside from reading our FunandFit.org blog, of course)?

❑ What's Really Being Defined?

One trick is to *check definitions and terms* before accepting the headline or sound bite. What is really being touted? In the aforementioned example, the article discussed the difference between long, slow, steady-state endurance exercise, compared with intervals of high- and mid-intensity cardio. The gist of the argument was that long-duration, low-intensity cardio doesn't train the heart to build resistance to stress. To reduce the risk of heart disease, we need to alternate intense exertion with active recovery periods.

Now, we're getting somewhere. We are *really comparing steady state cardio to high intensity interval training* (HIIT), relative to stress resistance. Two considerably different types of workouts. The low-and-slow cardio approach was once crowned queen of all "fat-burning zones," which has been rightly sent to the "dying myth zone." Certainly, a ton of studies and headlines have courted the new ruler, HIIT. "(HI) It's alive!" But, is the former type really "dead?" Or, as the participants in our group-fitness classes say, *"Just tell me what I am supposed to do. Is low-intensity cardio out and high-intensity now in?"*

❑ What Are Your Goals?

Sticking with this example, *why do you do cardio workouts in the first place?* To lose weight? To reduce menopause symptoms? To complete a half marathon? To avoid those darn heart attacks that run in your family? To climb to the top of Downton Abbey as you travel the world? To chase (and catch) Daniel Craig?

Your particular, personal, prioritized goals will guide you through the maze of confusing headlines. For example, your top goal may be to lose weight for an upcoming trip. In that scenario, high-intensity cardio might be your best choice, while the low, slow cardio needs to retire before you do. But, what if one of your high priorities is to stay cognitively aware and sharp as long as possible? Then, low-intensity cardio is *not* dead and may be what keeps you sharp, as you live longer and smarter. For brain boosting, casual cardio rules! Long live cardio! For the pounds-away program, long live the other cardio!

Can you see why you have to be willing to spend a little time and attention, when faced with the latest and faddiest media bites? Tempting as it is to believe headlines, the juicy bits are in the details: what's really being discussed (definition of terms) and who is this news really for (goal dependent)?

If you remember nothing else, just get out there and move. No matter your intensity, type of aerobic activity, or goals, you'll be better off. There we said it! Boom! Bonus tip: You'll also be better off if you sashay over to our blog to subscribe: Fun and Fit: Active Aging Answers for Boom Chicka Boomers (FunandFit.org).

Alexandra Williams, MA, has been in the fitness industry for over 30 years. Certified by the American Council on Exercise since 1986, she currently teaches in the exercise studies department at UC Santa Barbara, and is also an editor and a published writer for numerous magazines. In addition to sharing the blog FunAndFit.org: Active Aging Answers for Boom Chicka Boomers, with her identical twin sister Kymberly, Alexandra presents at numerous conferences throughout the U.S. Her advanced degree is in systemic counseling.

Kymberly Williams-Evans, MA, has taught fitness to more than 30,000 participants on 4 continents in four languages for more than three decades. Her career spans land, sea, and airwaves. Formerly a faculty member at UCSB in the departments of both exercise and sports studies and English, Kymberly has put her master's degree in English to good use, publishing articles, co-writing the fitness advice blog— www.FunandFit.org, speaking at events, and serving as inaugural editor for a professional publication. She teaches exercise classes in Santa Barbara, CA, where she continues to encourage people to reap the innumerable benefits of human movement.

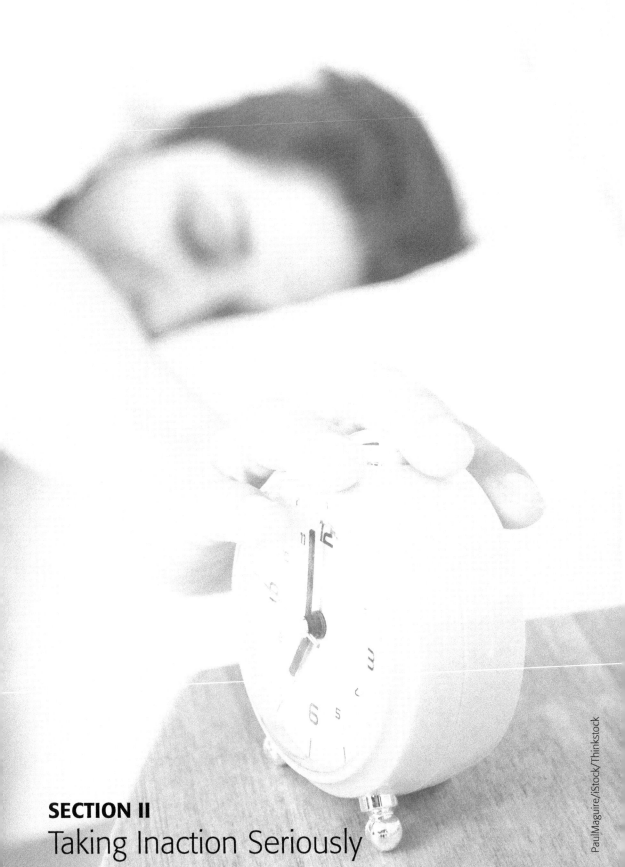

SECTION II
Taking Inaction Seriously

A good laugh and a long sleep are the best cures in the doctor's book.

—Irish Proverb

CHAPTER 5
Sleep Yourself Skinny

There really is a way to passively improve weight loss. What if all you had to do to lose weight was sleep more? Recent studies support this dream of getting slim passively. There's growing evidence that longer sleepers (compared to individuals who don't sleep nearly as long) are slimmer, with lower body mass index (BMI) levels, and perform better. Whether your chosen activity is golf, a triathlon, or mastering a sequence in Zumba, performance matters. Even if your game is getting to work and organizing dinner for the family clan, performance matters.

In spite of exercise and diets that should result in weight loss, your body could actually conserve your fat, at the expense of your lean muscle, without the right amount of shuteye. One study compared participants who slept 8.5 hours a night with individuals who slept 5.5 hours a night. The 5.5-hour group lost 55 percent less body fat and 60 percent *more* fat-free mass. Their metabolic hormone levels were also less favorable. Figure 5-1 details the relationship between sleep and hormones. One specific hormone, cortisol, is high when the amount of sleep is low. In other words, when the time you spend sleeping is relatively low, you're not only more likely to have cravings, you're also more primed to store calories as fat.

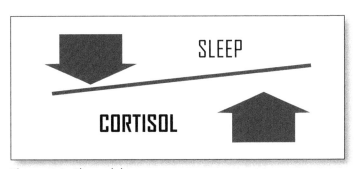

Figure 5-1. Sleep debt

Successful weight and body fat loss in short (i.e., seven hours or less) and average (i.e., seven to nine hours) sleepers improved when individuals increased their amount of sleep. Long sleepers (nine or more hours) didn't improve weight loss during the study. Such a result offers proof that while adequate sleep can optimize your weight and fat loss efforts, more than adequate isn't better. Getting more sleep boosted weight loss success by 33 percent only in those individuals who needed it.

Since sleep affects every aspect of life, it's important to be aware of the fact that not only does sleep duration enhance your weight *and* your weight loss efforts, exercise also benefits the quality of your sleep. It's a two-way street. It may not take a lot to improve your sleep. In fact, as little as 10 minutes of exercise a day can boost self-reports of sleep quality by nearly 30 percent.

A chronic lack of sleep alters hormones in the blood that control appetite and promote weight gain. Your sleep-deprived brain gets more signals to eat and fewer signals that you're full or satisfied. Too little sleep leads to changes in hunger and satiety hormones (ghrelin and leptin), which then signal the body to store excess energy. One study found that women maintained their weight during adequate sleep, whereas insufficient sleep reduces the dietary restraint and leads to weight gain in women.

HOW MUCH IS ENOUGH?

Most adults get about 6.5 hours of sleep a night. Optimal sleep recommendations vary by organization. In fact, this factor is such a grey area that the American Academy of Sleep Medicine, the Sleep Research Society, and Centers for Disease Control recently teamed to create new guidelines for sleep to include gender and age-specific guidelines.

Research findings about the amount of optimal sleep also vary, but agree on its importance. Currently guidelines recommend seven to nine hours of sleep for adults 50 to 70. A study at the University of California, San Diego, which tracked 1.1 million people over six years, showed a lower mortality rate among subjects who slept 6.5 to 7.4 hours a night; compared to those individuals who slept more or less.

Extended sleep can also result in lower energy. In addition, too long in bed was also associated with heart disease and diabetes. In another study, seven to eight hours of sleep were associated with an optimal level of body mass index (BMI). Seven hours seems to be the new eight.

There appears to be a gender difference in sleep needs, suggesting that women require more sleep, though in traditional roles they get less. Sleep is the time when your brain, as well as your body, recovers and "locks in" information that was processed during the day. If you're a woman who tends to multitask, or if you have a complex job with a lot of decision-making, you require even more sleep.

You'll soon find out how much sleep helps you personally function best. For now, know that accumulating sleep debt is a *big fat problem*.

How well can you exercise or make good food choices when you're drunk? A study of people deprived of sleep showed just two hours of sleep deprivation (sleeping six hours when you're used to eight) is similar to drinking two or three beers. In other words, if you lose four hours of sleep, it's the equivalent of having a 0.1 blood alcohol content level. Lose more sleep: operate more like you're drunk.

Besides putting the brakes on your weight loss, inadequate sleep means you lose lean muscle due to the missed opportunity to repair or rebuild muscles after exercise. Human growth hormone (HGH) is released most during deep sleep. HGH improves your level of fitness and performance, boosts protein synthesis, and facilitates the optimal recovery of muscle.

So, you can be exercising, and eating right, and still not get the desired results, without enough sleep. It would be a major challenge for you to lose fat weight or improve your level of fitness with an inadequate level of sleep.

How much sleep can you afford? How much can you afford to lose? What's the cost:benefit ratio? In our busy world, we look for "hacks" everywhere: ways we can do less and get the same or better results. The assumption is made that those individuals who can "get by" with a relatively few hours of sleep can get more done. That's not a reality for most people.

Separate research studies on collegiate swimmers, basketball players, and football players showed that extending the time of sleep beyond a normal level—up to 10 hours— led to significantly enhanced performance. Athletes were faster, had greater accuracy, and reported less daytime drowsiness and fatigue after both games and practice.

So, even if you're not an athlete or in college, you will undoubtedly reach a higher level of fitness by engaging in a higher *quality* of exercise, a scenario that's not going to happen sleepwalking. You're also more likely to exercise when you aren't already feeling tired or drained during the day. Fully rested, you're going to perform the desired exercise repetitions, complete your intervals, and achieve the heart rate response you want. Furthermore, if young college athletes at their peak of muscle mass can increase their level of performance with more sleep, there's a good chance you can also.

Simply getting 60 to 120 minutes more of quality sleep could improve your fat weight loss and fitness goals. As such, your question shouldn't be *whether* you need more sleep, it should be how do you get more and *how* much more exactly?

YOUR SLEEP NUMBER

First, determine your personal optimal sleep need. You'll find a helpful sleep needs worksheet in Appendix A-5.

Devote at least three days, and as much as a week, to a sleep needs experiment. Pick a three-day weekend or a vacation period during which you could ditch your alarm clock. Go to bed when you're tired and wake naturally. Record your total sleep time. At that point, you should have a good idea of your optimal sleep average.

Next, compare your optimal sleep average to what you're usually getting. If you've got a big gap, try to add half an hour a week to your sleep total. For most people, going to bed that much earlier can take some adaptation. It will feel too early. Give yourself the chance to see if you need the sleep. If you need an added incentive, be aware that an inadequate level of rest accelerates skin aging. Just saying.

At this point, look at the activities in your life you can limit or delete to close your gap. Internet surfing, TV, or reading might have to go. Can you change the time when you start work or find a way to reduce your commute to increase the amount of time you can spend in the sack?

Last, and biggest, is the challenge of knowing you need to and want to, *how* can you get the sleep? If you're one of the millions of people who have trouble falling asleep or staying asleep, helpful sleep tips are not new to you. Even if you've tried them all, refer to the section on pillow-talk tips and see if there might be even one thing that would be helpful to you.

NEED A SLEEP AID?

Sleeping naturally is best. Doctors agree sleeping without the aid of a drug is a higher quality sleep. There are ways you can help yourself naturally get more sleep. For example, magnesium may help calm and relax you. As such, find a citrate malate supplement and take it at night with your evening meal.

Another way to increase your magnesium levels is to soak in an Epsom salt bath. Among the symptoms of a magnesium deficiency are anxiety, insomnia, and muscle cramps. If you take a hot bath to help you sleep, you want to soak for at least 90 minutes before bed, so your temperature begins to drop, when you want to call it a night. Levels of magnesium can increase with two to three soaks a week. Just lock yourself in the bathroom, and tell the world you're busy.

Melatonin is a sleep-enhancing hormone, whose natural production is reduced with age. Exposure to sunlight in the morning can help in this regard. You may also want to try taking a melatonin supplement 90 minutes before bedtime. Timing makes a significant difference in melatonin's effectiveness. If all else fails, talk to your doctor about the pros and cons of sleep aids.

PILLOW-TALK TIPS

If you're exhausted, don't throw in the towel. Exhaust the following list first. Diligently, one-by-one, try them all. Don't expect months, years, or decades of poor sleep to disappear overnight (pun intended). Stick with the habits that help you sleep better for at least several weeks, before you decide what exactly works for you. Seek better, not perfect, sleep.

- Limit your caffeine to the morning hours; call it quits by 10 a.m. The Sleep Doctor allows more time for caffeine if this is a big leap. Take his recommendation at the end of this chapter first. Wean yourself gradually. If you experience better sleep, you can have your caffeine and sweet dreams too!
- Limit your intake of alcohol or eliminate it entirely.
- Quit using tobacco.
- Avoid "screen time" 90 minutes before bed. LED light (cell phone, computers, TV) signals the brain to stay awake. Keep your lights dimmer and at least 14 inches from your face in the evening.
- Set the room temperatures lower in the evening at 65 to 68 F. Cooler temperatures prepare your body for sleep.
- Take a hot bath or shower 90 minutes before bedtime. Your falling body temperature afterwards cues your body to sleep.
- Keep everything but sleep, sex, and your bedtime reading somewhere else.
- If you nap, keep your 15- to 20-minute nap to the early afternoon.
- Keep a diary of sleep quality and quantity, including any important details, like stressors, illness, and what you ate or whether you exercised.
- Keep a "worry" journal by your bed to write down your to-do list for tomorrow and anything you might otherwise stare at the ceiling thinking about later.
- Try a gratitude journal to begin and end your day on a positive note.
- Leave two to three hours between your last meal and bedtime. Don't go to bed hungry, however. A simple protein shake or a few almonds before bedtime are good choices, in this regard.
- Eliminate noise with earplugs or a white-noise machine.
- Create a dark environment, with either window fixtures or an eye mask.
- Invest in the best mattress, sheets, pillows, and pajamas that your money can buy.
- Use a reliable alarm clock (without an LED light pointed at you), so you're not worried about waking up in time.
- If you don't fall asleep within 30 minutes, get up and read or do something (no screen time), until you fall asleep.
- Establish a bedtime routine and stick to it. Create sleep cues, like removing make-up, taking a bath, dimming the lights, reading a few pages from a book, etc. Set a consistent time to go to bed and rise from bed.
- Get some sunlight early during the day and limit the level of artificial light after dark to boost your level of melatonin. This sleep-regulating production of hormones decreases with age. Try stimulating it naturally, and then talk to a doctor about supplements or other sleep solutions if you don't have success. If sleep apnea is suspected, a sleep lab stay can confirm whether it exists and suggest a viable treatment option that might bust your fat-loss plateau.

- Last, but not least, get some exercise. Even if you're sleep-deprived, a small dose of exercise is better than none. If you keep your exercise efforts to early in the day, it won't interfere with you settling down for a good sleep.

Your sleep needs might change from decade to decade. The following questions will help you decide if you're getting too much, too little, or just the right amount of dreamtime:
- Do you wake naturally?
- Do you wake feeling rested?
- Do you fall asleep easily?

In reality, if you're jolted out of sleep by an alarm clock, chances are you're not getting enough fat-loss-enhancing sleep.

You can't "catch up" easily. If you have a bad night's sleep or get to bed late, it's best to keep your usual wake-up time. Your biological clock will fare better getting right back on track, so you can fall asleep the next night on time or earlier, if necessary, to make up your debt.

Sleep is individual. Recommended guidelines target average needs for physical and cognitive health. Your body is the best gage. You'll wake when you've had enough.

FEATURED EXPERT

Dr. Michael Breus, The Sleep Doctor

❏ Five Steps to Better Sleep From the Sleep Doctor

Dr. Breus shares five steps you can take in order to help you get a better night's sleep and help yourself lose weight:

#1—Keep to one schedule. Going to bed at the same time and waking up at the same time, even on the weekends, turns out to be the most critical thing that you can do. So, if you get up at 6 a.m. during the week, you need to get up at 6 a.m. on the weekend. Even if you're out late partying until 3 a.m. in the morning, you want to get up and to do your thing during the day. In fact, it's going to be a very big obstacle for you if you don't. You want to go to bed at the same time and wake up at the same time every day.

#2—Eliminate caffeine by 2 p.m. Caffeine has a half-life of between 8 and 10 hours, which you may not know. You may say, "Oh, I can fall asleep after having had a big cup of coffee, and it's not a big deal." Well, the truth of the matter is that while you may be falling asleep, it is probably because you're so sleep-deprived. In fact, if you had EEG electrodes on your head, what you would discover is that you are, in fact, not getting a quality sleep. Caffeine kicks you out of the state of the deeper stages of sleep. So, stop caffeine by 2 p.m.

#3—Stop drinking alcohol three hours before lights out. As such, it takes the average human body approximately one hour per alcoholic beverage to be able to digest that alcoholic beverage. You may think that alcohol helps you fall asleep. In fact, it can make you feel sleepy. However, it keeps you out of the deep stages of sleep. As a result, the sleep that you get is very unrefreshing, which can lead to more sleep deprivation. So, stopping alcohol three hours before bed is the way to go.

#4—Stop any exercising about four hours before bed. Substantial evidence supports the fact that you should be exercising on a fairly regular basis. On the other hand, there is data that suggests that there are certain people who, when they exercise within that four-hour time frame before going to bed, are actually revved up, rather than being calmed down. Exercising too close to your bedtime can make it much more difficult for you to fall asleep, thanks to core temperature changes that prevent melatonin production.

#5—Get at least 15 minutes of sunlight every single morning, right after you wake up. Sunlight helps reset your circadian clock, and it's very, very, important for overall circadian health. Your biological clock runs half of your sleep cycle, and your sleep drive runs the other half. By getting sunlight in the morning, you will absolutely make sure that you can go to sleep and wake up when you need to.

Michael Breus, PhD, D,ABSM, aka The Sleep Doctor, is a clinical psychologist, board-certified in clinical sleep disorders. He is the sleep expert on WebMD and Sharecare. He also appears regularly on national television, including The Dr. Oz Show, The Doctors, *and* The Rachael Ray Show. *Furthermore, he provides expert advice and guidance in several leading national publications and websites, like* The Huffington Post. *He lives in Scottsdale, AZ. For more information, visit www. secretstosleepsuccess.com for* 10 Things Great Sleepers Do.

It's not stress that kills us, it's our reaction to it.

—Hans Selye

CHAPTER 6
The Stress Less Myth

Aging is not for the meek. Laughter is recommended for stress. Yet, you laugh too hard these days, and you wet yourself. Or pass gas. As a result, you need more laughter to get over the stress of the laughter. It's a vicious cycle.

Dr. Pamela Peeke's book, Fight Fat After Forty, which was published in 2000, was a landmark follow-up to her 1998 Shape Magazine article. It was at that point, that many individuals began to study the effects of stress on weight gain. Peeke had observed stress-induced weight occurring in individuals who weren't overweight.

Women over 40 are of particular risk due to hormonal changes occurring at the same time as certain life-stressors, such as caregiving, careers, and the difficulty prioritizing their own needs. As such, stress and hormones affected by stress are major culprits in the development of obesity. Stress management could provide the change you need for weight-loss success.

In 2011, the American Psychological Association conducted a survey on stress that revealed that nearly a quarter of Americans report stress levels are "extreme." In a similar survey, the average stress level was 5.1 on a scale of 10. While two-thirds of Americans are trying to reduce their level of stress, only one-third feel successful. Respondents agreed that stress has a negative impact on their quality of life. Furthermore, the study found that most women can easily identify with what stress feels like. Yet, nearly a third of those surveyed said that they believe stress is strictly psychological and has no impact on their physical health. Wrong. For your information, it is known that at least 80 diseases can be directly linked to stress.

Your first stress goal should be to reduce your overall exposure to chronic stress. As if emotional stress weren't enough, you're also exposed to environmental stressors all day in doses larger than ever before. The accumulation of toxins in your body means that your body will create new fat cells and store more toxins and fat within them. It's your body's way of protecting you by getting toxins out of circulation. Unfortunately, it also makes weight loss harder until this toxic problem is solved.

Visceral fat, i.e., deep abdominal fat, is affected equally by unhealthy eating, unhealthy activity, and chronic uncontrolled stress. Studies have found that relaxation techniques can reduce levels of cortisol in subjects. Accordingly, knowing that cortisol can block weight loss, five minutes of some chill would be a good investment.

If you're feeling out of control in other areas of life, when it comes to weight loss or even mood and energy, you probably tend to reach for tangible fixes initially. The intangible quality of stress reduction isn't measured as easily, as are minutes on a treadmill or pounds on a scale. While you can choose to reduce calories (though remember it doesn't have the effect you think it does), deciding to reduce your level of stress isn't nearly as easy. On the other hand, be forewarned that thinking this step is any less important than reducing your caloric intake is a mistake.

THE OTHER STRESS SOURCES

Toxins in your food, water, and air add stress to your body. They're hidden in several sources, including:

- Plastics made with bisphenol A (PBA)
- Cosmetics
- Lotions
- Perfumes
- Body and hair cleansers
- Cleaning products
- Nail products and salons
- Pesticides
- Teflon/aluminum pans
- Fire retardant materials
- Lawn and garden chemicals
- Dry cleaning products
- Heating and A/C
- Chlorine in pools
- Car exhaust
- Lead paint
- Mercury in certain fish (refer to Appendix B-4)
- Fluoride in water, toothpaste
- LED—"blue light"
- Furniture protectant

Some of these toxin-laden sources are directly linked to specific diseases. It's no secret that stress is a common denominator in every modern disease. It's difficult to measure your toxicity level. Pay attention to your body's signs, behavior changes, eating patterns, and signs of addiction. Such indicators don't have to be your normal.

Many of the signs of toxicity and stress you probably either accept as signs of age or confuse with many potential conditions. Fatigue, slowed metabolism, low motivation, constipation or diarrhea, and gas and bloating are symptoms that many women put up with on a daily basis.

Some people going through weight loss feel irritable, even on a reasonable caloric intake of healthy food. In part, this feeling is due to toxins being released into their blood. The more overweight you are, the more toxins you've stored. As toxins in the blood go up during weight loss, your levels of thyroid hormone go down. Your body has to be working as optimally as possible to deal with this situation.

Fiber acts like a sponge for your toxins. Fiber recommendations for women are 25 grams daily before age 50 and 21 grams thereafter. (Men should eat 38 grams daily before 50 and 30 after.) Yet, doctors and nutritionists suggest 35 to 50 grams per day, using supplemental fiber to ensure your levels are met. If you have a toxic issue, you might do best in the upper range. Check your fiber intake currently and if you've hit a plateau in weight loss, gradually increase your intake of fiber by five grams a week and see how you do.

Increase your awareness of stress symptoms in your body and mind. While this may seem obvious, women, especially, have adapted to a number of symptoms as "normal." Stress is unique to you. Your stress-related symptoms might include sleeplessness, tension, headaches, stomachaches, skin rashes, or acne. This list is by no means complete. You might be forgetful, unable to concentrate, or simply not be yourself. Some clients are frequently ill or suffer an increased level of injuries when they're under stress. The reason why they're encountering such circumstances, however, isn't obvious to them. Understand that you may not feel stressed. You may think you can handle it. If your body isn't responding positively to all the right lifestyle choices, though, it's telling you it's stressed!

If what stresses you is unique, and how it manifests itself in you is unique, it makes sense that your stress prevention kit will also have to be unique. There are, however, common steps that can help reduce stress or reduce the chance stress will sabotage your level of health and fitness, including the following:

- Plan ahead. Under stress, you are much more vulnerable to foods that don't serve your long-term goals. Avoid refined sugar. Focus on single servings. Eat early in the day. Eat mindfully, not on-the-go. Include high-quality fruits and vegetables and lean protein three to four times a day. When you're not stressed, put some meals in the freezer so you can effortlessly eat well under stress.
- Maintain the frequency of physical activity. Even though it's often first to go, don't dump exercising completely. Have a regular routine, as well as a routine under stress. If you're recovering from a lack of sleep, reduce either the duration or the level of intensity of your exercise, or both. If you're mentally distracted, ride an exercise bike instead of riding the road.

Work, relationships, finances, exercise, and diet are all potential sources of stress. Your body and mind don't separate them. Your being is dealing with the entire allostatic load. Imagine yourself walking up two flights of stairs. You know what that feels like. OK, now imagine you are carrying a full laundry basket. That represents your work stress.

A few steps up, you have to put on a backpack full of bricks. Hypothetically, that scenario is a close family member diagnosed with a chronic health condition. Up a few more steps are big books that you pile on the laundry. That's the extreme-exercise and low-calorie diet you're on this week to lose weight.

By now, you're straining to take a step, and you're off-balance. Instead of making it to the top, you sit down, stuck halfway up. You have to put something down in order to make the trip. What do you need to put down?

Stress is affecting your hormones and putting breaks on weight loss efforts, no matter how little you eat and how much you exercise. That combination, in fact, could make weight loss harder, not easier.

You may have begun to accept the logic, somewhere along the way, that exercise and diet are punishment. As such, exercising and dieting have to be uncomfortable, hard, and hurt, or leave you hungry, tired, and irritable. When you approach the two activities that way, you contribute more to the release of negative stress hormones that push you further from achieving permanent weight loss and optimal health.

If you still refer to exercise as an optional part of your life, there's a strong chance that you'll always struggle. Without question, exercise is mandatory. You were meant to move. Motion drives emotion. If you are carrying a basket of stressors, you need to find movement that gives you joy. It is your key. Trying to blast fat off of you by overzealous exercise is going to either make you hate it, or backfire by causing a negative stress response in your body.

Stress in your body is often referred to as inflammation. It's a natural response to protect and repair constant exposure to toxins. If this response is turned on all the time, your system's allostatic load is more than you can carry. It is also an obstacle to successfully reaching a healthy weight or fitness level.

Stress, whether from a job that exposes you to chemicals, from your own irrational thoughts (everyone has them), or from a mismatched diet and exercise plan, causes higher metabolic rates, adrenalin, and cortisol that then speed up the acidifying process. Though a higher metabolic rate might sound good, you can't have that and not all the rest as a stress response. On top of that, if you tend to reach for coffee, sugar, dairy, meat, "junk," or processed foods that cause nutrient deficiency, your liver will struggle. More stress.

When your system's crucial internal organs aren't functioning well, weight loss is going to be a challenge. If you can't see under the hood, what do you do?

Adding specific nutrients back into your diet and balancing your system with more inflammation-stopping foods may make a major difference. Load your diet with anti-inflammatory nutrients that can be easily absorbed. Balance your omega 6 fats, which flip the inflammation switch on, with your intake of omega 3 fats that flip inflammation off. In addition, keep in mind that your toxic thoughts and relationships can stress your body as much as toxic chemicals in your food, water, and air do.

YOUR STRESS RX

What is the best medicine? Is it laughter? It might be. Positive chemistry reactions in the body occur with deep belly laughter. What makes you laugh is unique. It is likely that your chances of laughing are much higher around people, than if you're alone. Accordingly, feed your need for laughter with your friends and colleagues. In addition to laughter, every single stress-reducer on the following list has a body of research showing reductions of physiological stress responses in the body:

- Exercising
- Journaling
- Learning or hobbies
- Massage, steam, baths
- Meditation and spirituality
- Mindless activities
- Music
- Nature
- Pets
- Social connectivity
- Yoga, deep breathing, progressive relaxation

STRESS RESIDUE

Stress knots the stomach and makes your head pound. Tension causes pain in the neck, extending to your upper back and shoulders, which is where many women carry the weight of the world. Massage therapists say they can predict the occupations of clients by where they carry their stress. Audiences composed of primarily women asked whether they have tight shoulders or neck issues will result in about 90 percent of the heads in the room nodding. Men, on the other hand, have a greater tendency to carry their stress in their lower back.

Chances are you are much more comfortable with tangible control, as opposed to esoteric stress reduction. You seek exercise and diet changes, before considering intangible and complex changes in your relationships and emotions. If you feel like you have less control in other areas of your life, you're more likely to reach for more exercise and diet control.

Many weight loss-seeking clients report a recent history of unexplained and "coincidental" injuries. Overzealous exercise, or simply not following the exercise-under-stress plan, and assuming that you'll just push through it with discipline and willpower can sideline you, thereby creating further stress.

You can't rob Peter to pay Paul. It's so cliché, and sadly, so true. If you don't have the right nutritional support (or you're not absorbing it) or emotional support (or you're rejecting that), you can't exercise those gaps away. You can't outrun a poor diet, and you can't outrun a bad relationship or job. You need to remove toxins from your environment in as many ways as possible. Confront that relationship conflict at home or work. A little acute stress is much less costly to health than chronic long-term stress. Enhance your coping skills, so you actually get to the problem, not just the symptoms.

MORE HIDDEN STRESSORS

Over-the-counter and prescription drugs can stress the body. Sometimes, it can't be avoided. Yet, too much for too long of any drug can have side effects on other parts of your body as well.

Exercise is stress on the body. The right dose supports energy and positive emotion. The wrong dose can contribute to hormonal imbalance.

Diet is also stress on the body. A colleague said, "The body needs recovery from dieting." It's so true.

When you're feeling high levels of stress, your body responds with higher levels of cortisol in the brain. That's compounded by the fact that under stress, sleep is often disrupted. Remember, if the level of sleep is low, the level of cortisol is high. As a result, abdominal fat has more cells, as well as higher blood flow and more glucocorticoid receptors. The abdominal area provides a more welcoming, easier landing site for fat than your subcutaneous pinch-an-inch kind of fat on the upper arms or over the jeans does.

STRESS IS UNIQUE TO YOU

If cortisol is the belly-fat diva, oxytocin is the teddy bear or puppy. It's known as the cuddle-hormone. Oxytocin is released by social interactions. It protects the cardiovascular system and acts as an anti-inflammatory agent.

Two recent studies proved caring for other people or volunteering during periods of high stress may buffer the effects of your stress. Public records of survey participants, who said they were experiencing high stress, were checked after five years. In general, high stress resulted in higher-than-normal mortality rates, except in caregivers and volunteers. No increase in stress-related death among them occurred. While a caregiver's health is often a concern, it may be that their very act of nurturing others is their stress buffer.

It is important to remember that what stresses one person may not stress you. On the flip side, you've got to be aware of internal and external signs in your body, even something you enjoy, that may be causing you stress. You may not always recognize it. Orthorexia, though not an official mental disorder, is an unhealthy obsession with eating healthy food. Addiction to exercise to the point you do it when you're ill or injured is a stressor. While these two examples are extreme, your own under-the-radar-stressor can be much more mild and yet add to your total load of stress.

THE POWER OF STRESS MANAGEMENT

A recent study found that women in an eight-week weight loss program who also participated in stress management had a greater weight loss than those who did not participate in progressive relaxation and diaphragmatic breathing exercises.

In her TED Talk, Stanford University lecturer and health psychologist Kelly McGonigal talked about the new science of stress. According to McGonigal, it's not stress, but how you think about stress that's the problem. If you believe stress is making you stronger and more resilient, instead of believing it is bad for your health, you will live longer. Rethink your attitude toward stress.

The real answer to ending your stress-related weight might be to get more resilient. You're not going to get rid of or avoid stress. Across several studies, subjects who lived longer with stress found the answer: they got better at dealing with it. You can change the biology of stress in your body by the way you think about stress. If you think it's bad for your health and is making you fat, it will. For years, we've focused on countering the bad effects of stress. New thinking claims that there's a better way.

If you categorize your stress, you have good, tolerable, and toxic stress. Acute and intermittent (good) stressors boost your immune system. What falls in this category? Two examples of such stressors are a project due Friday or a short-interval workout.

Tolerable stress could be caring for someone for an extended period of time or studying for a tough test that you've selected, because it will improve your career. You do what you have to do. Once it's over, however, there's no irreversible damage.

When sustained or chronic stress becomes toxic, you feel an unrelenting stress that is traumatic, combined with a feeling of a lack of control or social support. You're isolated or feeling social rejection. An example of such a scenario could be a negative job situation without a light at the end of the tunnel or a chronic and an unpredictable health condition without a good prognosis.

While excess weight is stress on your body, including joints, heart, and your endocrine system, the way you think about your weight is also more stress. This factor is one that you can put under your control, which is not to suggest a love-your-fat fest. Yet, if harsh and strict methods of exercise and diet haven't worked, yoga or meditation will burn the fewest calories, but could reach your fat-causing stress faster than high-intensity interval hell.

Brian Luke Seaward

❑ Stress Strategy: Six Steps for Stress Success

- #1. Move from fear to love. Change can bring fear motivated stress behavior. Living in these times of rapid change as we are, people tend to stay engaged in the stress response. Embrace change, knowing that something good always comes out of change. Focus on what better is waiting ahead.
- #2. Turn off the news. News and politics capitalize on fear.
- #3. Meditate. Resolve that the causes of stress are not the same as just the symptoms. Headaches and hemorrhoids get our attention. Finding the source of your stress is more difficult. Prolonged stress is about ego (control dramas). There is no medication to tame the ego.
- #4. Identify ineffective, stress-coping strategies in your life. Your ineffective strategies could include drinking, drugs, or inordinate amounts of time surfing the 'net. Replace these with effective stress management strategies that relax the body and help the mind cope with, rather than avoid, stress.
- #5. Stock your own stress toolbox. The more stress management tools you have in your toolbox, the more quickly you'll find resolution. You'll be able to choose an appropriate stress strategy for each specific stressor. In that regard, explore the following tools:
  - ✓ Reframing: shift from negative thinking to positive thinking
  - ✓ Humor
  - ✓ Time management
  - ✓ Creative problem solving
  - ✓ Journaling
  - ✓ Healthy boundaries
  - ✓ Art therapy
  - ✓ Dream therapy
  - ✓ Meditation
- #6. Use the examples of others to help find your own approach. My day, for example, begins with a walk in a nature preserve near my home. When I return I meditate for 30 to 40 minutes. I swim at noon. I play instrumental music in the background, while I work. I don't own a cell phone, and I turn off the WiFi router at 8 p.m. I enjoy some comic relief, and a monthly massage, as well as regular time with friends and my dog. I know quality alone time clears my head. Meditation has been powerful for me. I do fairly well, including daily stress-coping strategies. What will you include in your stress strategy?

Brian Luke Seaward, PhD, is the author of the bestselling books, Stand Like Mountain, Flow Like Water; Stressed Is Desserts Spelled Backward; *and* The Art of Calm. *He is the executive director of the Paramount Wellness Institute in Boulder, CO, and can be reached at www.brianlukeseaward.net.*

The body needs to rest. It needs a lot less exercise than you think.

CHAPTER 7 ——————————————
Rest Your Way to Best

R&R is important. That's not suggesting twin La-Z-Boy recliners. If you want to end jumping off the bed to get your pants on *and* snapped though, you might … wait for it … consider doing less. By some mean-girl freak-of-nature just when you thought you had it figured out—i.e., I work hard, I get better results—someone went and changed the rules.

Yes, you need to move frequently. Yes, when people say *just do it* most days a week, they're right. Is it right *for you*, right now the right question? If what you're doing isn't working, the answer usually is *not* to do *more* of it.

Does it feel like you're drowning between planning meals, exercising, working, and undertaking life's to-do lists? Add the occasional extra project, as well as the chance you might have a friend or relationship, and you're in constant motion. When was the last time you planned to rest?

"I don't work that hard. I don't need a day off." If you've ever said that, stop it. It's exactly the point. When you don't rest, everything becomes grey. You don't have any hard days, easy days, moderate days, and days off. You probably take the same approach during exercise. Instead of intervals and recovery periods, it all blends together at about the same level of intensity all of the time. Your fitness level suffers. Your system suffers. Your chance of losing weight suffers.

Any exercise program can make you tired, or bored. The one you'll stick with will challenge you some days and let you off easy on others. It will reward you with better hormone health, mood, and optimal weight, without depriving, exhausting, or injuring you.

There are half a dozen ways to look at rest and recovery. Buckle your seatbelt. You're going to get a glimpse at them all. Initially, you'll see how within a workout, rest requires thought. Then, from one day to the next and the week overall, there's the artful orchestration of work and recovery dancing with each other. Left to chance, someone could get her toes stepped on.

If you were raised to believe that the harder you work, the better results you get, taking your rest will be hard. Jennifer believed working harder would get her better results. She enjoyed working hard and feeling like she'd done her best. At 62, though, she suffered two injuries within two years that sidelined her. At one point, she had complete rest and at another point was forced to minimize her level of activity. The inactivity was more painful for Jennifer than the injury itself. Once she was able to resume exercising, she began to take one day off a week. Now, she rests two full days a week and has light recovery days when she needs those too. She's got more energy, as well as fewer illnesses and injuries to show for it.

You may have ignored the need for recovery until now. You want results, and you want them yesterday. It's easy to forget the basics of exercise. The fundamental point is that the real progress you achieve by exercising, i.e., gaining strength, increasing muscle, and elevating metabolism, occurs *between* workouts.

Quick recovery, after a challenging workout, is one of the underlying factors that is essential to successful weight loss. If you are someone who likes exercise and wants to exercise frequently, you need to be recovered. The sooner you are recovered, the sooner you can do another workout and gain from it. The more hard work you can do in a given amount of time, the more fit you become. The key is quick recovery. If you're not recovered and attempt another punishing workout, you go backward, instead of forward.

Have you taken a multi-day-per-week extreme boot camp and found yourself much more fatigued by Thursday or Friday? Have you found small signs of injuries after several weeks of building intensity? Did you experience illness just after or during an intense program? Such signs do not necessarily indicate that the exercise was bad, but rather that the recovery wasn't adequate.

If you don't love exercise, you may not be chomping at the bit to work out again. Even so, you still want to recover quickly. Your efforts to fire on all cylinders to end your brain fog, boost your energy level, or lose weight depend on it. Neglect recovery, and your muscles break down, and your hormones *par-tay*. Need for recovery from exercise is increasingly important, if you're unduly stressed, even if your schedule is tight.

A new workout deliberately damages your muscle tissue, causing a short-term reduction in strength, speed, and oxygen delivery. Inflammation and immune system hormones and chemicals begin circulating to minimize and repair the damage. Swelling and muscle soreness complete the process. So, even if you're a superwoman, you still need to recover from the demands you place on your body.

Are you convinced you need recovery to find optimal energy and weight management yet? If yes, then your question is how do you recover? What if you can't lie around eating avocados (with protein, of course) and getting a massage after a workout?

Is recovery one day or two? How does nutrition content and timing boost recovery? How do you balance recovery with your weight-loss goals? What's best for you—complete rest or light activity? If active recovery is best, which type? You'll get answers to all those questions in upcoming sections of this chapter.

Everybody's physiology recovers differently from workouts and from stressors. One study found that it took between 5 and 89 days for different participants to return to full strength after an intensive weight-training program, which indicates how different individuals can be.

Other research that measured recovery from a three-week period of intensive training found that two weeks of recovery benefited one-third of the participants tremendously, another third moderately, and another third not at all. Getting feedback so you know if you're recovered or not can mean the difference between exercise that moves you toward your goal and exercise that's standing between you and your goal.

If you're a woman on a mission to lose weight, you can get blindsided by not understanding that the stressors in your life affect the level of your fitness. If you're depressed, stressed, or feel messed with, your recovery from exercise is different than when you're all que sera, sera. Your system could already be stressed from non-exercise stressors. It matters.

You might need recovery every day just *from* the every day. If you're seriously stressed about work, your financial status, a certain colleague's personality, or the fact that your boss is a tyrant, you've got physical stress emanating from it. You don't even have to go for the workout to elevate your heart rate, cortisol, and adrenaline. You're physically worked over. Guess what? Your body doesn't know the difference.

At this point in your life, you may feel older and wiser. Then again, you may just feel older. A late-in-the-day exercise class, when your cortisol levels are dropping, is not your best option. Yoga or a soothing stroll outdoors and unplugged may be just the workout you need.

The point to remember is that a workout can *be* recovery or it can *require* recovery. You want to start planning your exercise stressors with your life stressors in a way that exercise makes you better, not just tired. You want both the highs and lows, the challenging and the easy.

The question isn't whether a class, an instructor, or a DVD is "good" or bad. It's whether it's good for you at a particular point in your life. In fact, ask whether it's good for you at the time of day it's offered. If you're already highly stressed and not sleeping well, a late-day high-intensity exercise class could push you further out of balance and away from your skinny jeans. If you aren't getting signs you're full after you've eaten plenty, late-day intervals, on the other hand, could be exactly the right answer. You don't need what your best friend needs, even though that might be fun. You need what your hormones need right now.

A fascinating comparison of two studies on training intensities of cyclists showed different results from similar training. Right, I know you may not be a pro cyclist, but bear with me and imagine the tight bike shorts. One study done in 2002 and another in 2010 used similar training conditions to impose overtraining on the subjects. In other words, they made them do far more and at higher intensities than they were used to. In the first study, the performance level of the athletes went down. In the second study, all of the same signs of overtraining existed, but this level of performance did not suffer. Why?

The only difference was that the second study was conducted in a camp-like setting. Think *Biggest Loser*. All of the subjects had to focus on was training, nutrition, and sleep. There were no everyday distractions or stressors. The basic point is that under ideal recovery conditions, your body can respond to and repair damage from intense training. Under real-life conditions, it is more likely that negative factors will inhibit your ability to recover.

Whether you're responding to a new level of intensity during a workout with your trainer, you're dieting for weight loss, or you're worrying about a personal problem, your brain's hypothalamic-pituitary-adrenal axis (HPA) acts on that pea under your mattress and produces adrenaline and cortisol among other hormones. These hormones increase your heart rate, process fuel, and begin repairing areas of your body that have been damaged by a stressor. It sounds like good news, at first glance.

What if you have all of those stressors going on at the same time? Your body has a harder time recovering. You need an exercise program that accounts for all of these challenges.

Knowing how much individual and situational variation exists in recovery should help soften the blow, if you see others attending the same exercise class or eating the same as you, who are getting great results, while you struggle. No two people have the same response to change.

If you go to the same boot camp as a friend, chances are you may be pushed and prodded and encouraged by peer pressure to do more … not just more than you think you can, but more than you potentially *should*, particularly if your body is just simply a slow-recovering vessel. It's not a sign of weakness. Rather, it's just a highly variable thing, and if you're following a boot-camp drill sergeant or trying to keep up with a friend, you could do less good and more harm than if you recover fully.

Gender recovery response varies too. Men and women suffer the same amount of muscle soreness after intensive weight lifting, but women have a lower inflammatory response. Interestingly, women still take longer to return to peak strength and range of motion.

For example, you and a male colleague (e.g., spouse or friend) do the same workout, with comparable work. You would have less inflammation, but in 48 hours, you may not be as strong at the consecutive workout as he will. You might do better on a Monday-Thursday schedule, while he can do well with a Monday-Wednesday schedule. In fact, there's quite a bit of research showing that most older adults do better with not one, but two, days between hard workouts.

The big message is listen to your body. Ignore the social memes that tell you pain is weakness leaving your body. On occasion, it's your body still recovering from the prior workout, and it shouldn't be pushed to do another one, until it's back to full strength.

If your cortisol levels are out of balance, it's time to reduce your level of activity—or at least plan it more carefully—and increase your level of nutrient density. Signs of cortisol roadblocks, which are discussed in more detail in Chapter 8, include afternoon cravings, poor sleep quality or quantity, and growing belly fat, contrary to your best efforts. Cutting back on exercise, though, can be hard.

Exercise for many women becomes a stress-coping mechanism. When it works, you can get carried away. It's easy to understand why. You start to exercise, feel better because of it, and keep it up. As you begin to enjoy the benefits of a trimmer waistline and more curves, you feel better about yourself. As a result, you're motivated to do more. Subsequently, if your exercise regimen becomes more intense, involves more minutes per session, and encompasses more days of the week … pretty soon, you're adding stress, instead of helping yourself cope with stress.

Without adequate rest and recovery to complement your exercise efforts, you will increase your level of cortisol and inflammation. The situation entails too much of a good thing, which can cause you to plateau. You stop seeing results, start feeling "flat" or tired, and derail your weight-loss efforts.

When you're faced with a lot of different stressors (e.g., work, family, and finances—all of which are compounded by exercise and too little rest or inadequate nutrition), your system can get caught in a stress hormone-inflammatory loop. Hormones are released at higher levels, which can lead to a pro-inflammatory response. As a result, more cortisol is present, which can increase your level of inflammation.

Your optimal exercise routine will optimize your cortisol and adrenaline levels. It stimulates endorphins—your natural painkillers and mood elevators.

Research indicates that high-intensity (> 70 percent of maximal effort) exercise sessions, lasting longer than 20 to 30 minutes, or low-intensity (< 50 percent to 70 percent) efforts, lasting longer than 75 minutes, can flood the body with stress and inflammation biochemical markers. As a result, the exact opposite of what you actually want occurs. A negative domino effect is initiated on all things involving weight loss and achieving a happy hormone balance. Exercising at less than the 70 percent effort level seems to be the baseline for reducing inflammation and stress hormone levels.

In other words, any conversations after an exercise class that start with *"how many calories did I just burn?"* lack common sense. If burning the most calories during a workout is your focus, you're ignoring the underlying hormone rules of weight loss. Weight loss is not just a matter of controlling calories in and calories out. Hormones control the keys to unlocking your sexy, post-50 selfie. If you try to burn the most calories every time you work out, there's a chance that you'll send your hormones running in the opposite direction from your desired weight loss goal. As a result, you'll be the one burned.

R&R NOW AND LATER

Exercise prescription should follow the FITT acronym. Your best recovery should adhere to the same planning measures: frequency, intensity, time, and type of activity and recovery. Doing so will have a positive impact on the results you achieve.

Your optimal level of fitness, leanness, and health start with a well-thought-out plan. Consider everything from day-to-day sessions to entire training cycles. For athletes, cycles define what they do during the pre-season, in-season, or off-season. For you, summer may be either your more active "in season" cycle (e.g., play your best golf), or when you want to look good sleeveless.

Your best fitness results start with a plan involving each of the following points of recovery:
- During a workout, between sets of weights or cardiovascular intervals
- During the day, between workouts morning and evening or same-day competitions
- Within your training week, between workouts
- Within longer training cycles of weeks and months

If you treat your body like it's your business (which it is), you'll start thinking in quarters. What is your focus for the next 90 days? Are you peaking for fun runs and races? Are you getting stronger for a better golf outing in the spring? Are you hoping to drop chins at your next class reunion?

Exercise routines that achieve the best results are planned, not accidental. The widely popular and results-driven interval training is a great example. When you begin your interval training, your intervals should be fewer in number and have an equal or longer recovery period. As you progress, the recovery period can either be reduced or the interval can be increased, or ultimately both. A good coach or instructor will change one major component at a time. If you're coaching yourself, you should do the same.

Using the aforementioned information, for example, your first interval endeavor might be 30 seconds, which is like running from one gate to the next in the airport or running back to the kitchen to get the kale chips before they burn. In reality, your life is filled with intervals. As such, your recovery period should be 30 seconds, 45 seconds, or more.

There's some evidence that exercise trends and fads can provide you with a lot of opportunity to get in trouble. For example, if you've tried the popular Tabata workouts or have had an excited instructor share her new weekend workshop workout with you, it's clear that progression is a missing ingredient when it comes to interval training. The research-based and popular Tabata intervals involve 20 seconds of high-intensity exercise and 10 seconds of recovery, repeated eight times over a four-minute period per set. You'll often do repeated sets in a class. This protocol is one that caters to individuals who are the most fit. As such, if you don't have a fitness foundation yet, hold off on Tabata.

The subjects in the research conducted by Tabata were elite cyclists who worked at 110 percent intensity during high intervals and who rested, while sitting on their bikes, between intervals. Neither of those variables would be recommended for an individual who is just starting to exercise by a responsible exercise physiologist who is liable for that person's well-being.

When appropriate, planned intervals can offer you a two-for-one. For example, some forms of interval training can help you recover better from exercise. The exercise isn't just helping you get fit; it's also helping your body train to be able to sweep nasty lactate and toxins that follow exercise out of your body better. The resultant balance of work and recovery naturally boosts your body's ability to get the break it needs to reduce cumulative damage from exercise.

Two-minute intervals, with one-minute periods of recovery, provided you're breathing pretty hard during your two-minute intervals, will boost your $\dot{V}O_2$max, which is a quantitative indicator of the volume of oxygen you can consume. It's a measure of fitness. The more fit you are, the higher your $\dot{V}O_2$, and the quicker you recover from your bout of exercise. When you're doing intervals, you need to be working at about 100 percent $\dot{V}O_2$max for the training effect to be most beneficial. That's not a comfortable place just off the couch. Relax, you'll get there.

Another and a more appropriate interval plan for getting off the couch is a 1:3 to 1:4 work:recovery ratio. In this plan, you perform short intervals of 30 seconds, followed by longer recovery of between 90 seconds to two minutes. You need to feel like you're engaged in an "all-out" sprint to the shoe sale at Nordstrom during the work interval. Look to Chapter 4 on movement matters for more details about how to start and progress your interval training. Progress—don't guess. You want specific, not random, results. As such, you need to avoid random acts of fitness.

One factor that is particularly risky about extreme boot camp formats is that while working hard for five to six days a week may be a type A's dream, it's also a potential hormone nightmare. One to three days a week of interval training, with at least 48 hours recovery between workouts, is optimal. Start with one day. Choose the program that best meets your needs. Too much too soon is, and always has been, a formula for injury. For the after 50 female, it's also a fat-belly formula. Your hormones don't need any help stressing. You can work hard. You just need to take it one hormone at a time.

Recovery rules for weight training are similar. The heavier you lift (i.e., the fewer repetitions), the more rest between sets and between days of lifting you want. If you're doing six to eight repetitions (as opposed to 15) you want two to three minutes of rest between sets. You could do something else during that time. To comply with normal gym etiquette (and if you want to make friends and influence others), don't sit on the leg press between your sets. Definitely don't sit on the leg press and check your phone messages. Instead, go do an upper-body exercise and then return to the leg press. You'll provide your working muscles with adequate rest between sets, without wasting more of your precious time.

If you're doing more repetitions with lighter weights, as you would do in circuit training (a regimen that has proven to be very effective at boosting strength, endurance, and aerobic capacity), you move from one exercise to the next with minimal rest between. The underlying premise of this approach involves the fact that by the time you circle back to repeat an exercise, your working muscles have gotten the required rest.

Previously, you read about choosing the right routine to achieve your goals in Chapter 4. Review the information in Chapter 4 if you're planning your exercise and recovery at this point. Ponder the thought that your recovery period is as important as the work itself, both within the workout and otherwise.

Recovery time also refers to time during your training day. For whatever reason, you might have to split your exercise efforts into cardio in the morning and strength training in the evening. Make sure you have at least six hours between the two split workouts and, if possible, plan optimal recovery strategies around those workouts. So, if you're rushing to the office from the gym, make sure you have some nutrition (i.e., foodstuffs) with you to boost your recovery. Get used to packing a cooler in the car for reasons other than attending a tailgate.

Your exercise regimen, during the week, should involve rotating hard and easy days that allow for recovery. Use your calendar to plan your week. If you end up having to be flexible when something comes up, make sure you look at changes to the week as a whole.

Training cycles should consider the big picture. You may not be training for a triathlon or a 5K, but if you're embarking on a life change, take eight- or 12-week blocks at a time. Within three months, you should incorporate three or four "recovery weeks" that are slightly lighter in intensity overall. Adaptations, never forget, occur during the rest and recovery from exercise.

RECOVERY WITHIN YOUR WEEK

How many days of high-intensity exercise can you do during a given week? The older you are, the fewer high intensity days you want for optimal fitness. It's best to exercise with intention at any age or fitness level. Avoid graying your workouts, along with the graying of your tresses, and you'll reach and keep a higher level of fitness.

In other words, if Monday is devoted to doing intervals, Tuesday could be earmarked for performing a longer, slower, steady workout. Don't be tempted to include intervals into every workout. It just makes everything cloudy. Determine a purpose for exercising and stick to it. Be sensitive to symptoms that tell you that you need more rest. If you've been exercising and not seeing results, it may indeed be your hormones, but it could also be that you haven't been exercising with a purpose.

As interval or strength workout intensities increase, the frequency of your workouts should decrease in order to avoid breaking down. You absolutely can work hard as you age. Keep in mind, however, you have to allow your body the opportunity to recover. You don't have a decreased capacity for work, as much as you have an increased need for recovery. It simply takes longer as you age. Fast intervals, heavy strength-building loads, or long bouts of exercise require additional recovery. If you're fatigued from your exercise routine, put several days between your "hard" sessions. Exercise, after all, is supposed to give you more energy and make you stronger. If these are not the results you're achieving, it's time to regroup.

Are you just getting off the couch? Maybe, you're just finding "you" time again. Make building a habit your focus. Exercising 20 minutes most days of the week is a good start. Next, when you've got a basic foundation of fitness, give each day more purpose by doing intervals one day and a longer endurance session another. Keep your other days short-to-moderate and try biking or spending time in the pool. Take a tip from healthy, older athletes, who cross-train, which is exercising, but using different levels of intensity and impact and different modes of exercise.

Take two days off exercise each week and be active in other activities in your life. When the intensity level of your workouts increases, the frequency of how often you exercise should go down and the amount of rest or the days you devote to recovery should increase. Doing more purposeful exercise on fewer days of the week leads to more gains in fitness, less fatigue, and fewer injuries. It's about quality, not quantity.

You don't have to be a football player to do two-a-day workouts. For many individuals, time is a big obstacle with regard to exercising. If that's true for you, split your exercise routine into cardio in the morning and strength later in the day, in order to solve your problem. Tend to adequate nutrition and rest between workouts.

TYPE OF EXERCISE AND NEED FOR RECOVERY

The type of exercise you do influences your need for recovery. Running, for example, is higher impact and more damaging to muscle tissue. High-intensity interval training requires at least 48 hours between workouts, even more when you're just starting out. Optimal recovery from heavy strength training for older adults is 72 hours.

Swimming, cycling, and rowing are examples of easier-on-the-body exercises. As such, a swim or an easy spin on a bike could be a recovery session. You might prefer to complement your cardio workouts with yoga or stretching instead. The point is that there are rules, and while they're important, you need to be flexible. Create a plan for each week. An example of such a plan is included in Chapter 4. Be sure to apply the way you feel, as well as any time constraints you may have, to your plan. Determine if you're giving recovery a chance to help you get lean and boost your energy level.

Functional exercise is frequently recommended to older adults. In reality, the term is somewhat elusive. All exercise is functional. Your goal should be to make your exercise efforts functional, relative to you. As a rule, functional exercise encompasses purposeful movement that focuses on balance, agility, and reaction skills. Many exercise professionals suggest that you move away from working out on stable exercise machines and spend more time performing movements that are similar to daily activities of living.

Fortunately, balance, agility, reaction, and coordination exercise requires less recovery and can be done more frequently. If you enjoy daily exercise, the right blend of balance and agility work, between heavier strength training days, will help you meet that goal. Strength exercises that increase bone density and lean muscle mass can either be alternated with more functional exercise days or done on the same day. Create a plan and then work the plan.

RECOVERY WEEKS

It's time to think about weeks as they relate to months at a time. Conscious planning will get you safely to your goal. In that regard, there are a few factors, however, that you need to consider. For example, you need to ascertain both the training variables (e.g., frequency, intensity, and duration) and components (e.g., strength, cardio, and flexibility) attendant to your exercise regimen and then insert this information into your calendar in the form of the activities you enjoy.

If you perform the same routine every week, your level of fitness will initially progress. Over time, however, it will plateau. You want to intentionally build and recover from fitness challenges. Remember that high-intensity or long workouts are "hard" days, while low-intensity spinning, swimming, or walking sessions are easy days. At this point, you should think about entire weeks as easy, moderate, or hard. When you look at the total volume and intensity of your workouts on a week-to-week basis, you can plan your expenditure of time and energy ahead. At first glance, it may sound complicated, but you're probably already doing this.

When you initially began to exercise, hopefully, you started with working out fewer days of the week or doing bouts of exercise that were shorter in duration, because you weren't as fit. Maybe, you went to an hour class but couldn't do all of it. You rested frequently.

All factors considered, as you get stronger and gain endurance, you can go further, do more repetitions, or last longer. Those changes occur over weeks and months. If you want to bump up your enjoyment of exercise and the level of results as you age, you'll think about how you piece together your exercise puzzle. If you belong to a fitness center with a wide variety of classes into which you can drop at time you want, you'll have to do more planning yourself. Those classes have a responsibility to offer the intensity described on the class schedule every time they're conducted. You need to think about what effort level you will need to give to be in accordance with your personal exercise plan (PEP).

If you enjoy competing in races, fun runs, or walks, you'll need additional recovery after an event. The added adrenaline and excitement can cause you to have more micro-tears in your muscles, even if you think you're not competitive! If you train for life experiences, like riding your bicycle across the state for a week or walking the Appalachian Trail or the Camino in Spain, your recovery might last several weeks following those big experiences. Your regimen is similar to an athlete. You work increasingly harder and train for the event. Then, you do the event. Finally, you need to rest.

Increase the level of intensity *or* the volume of your exercise efforts for three weeks, and then reduce the intensity, volume, and frequency of your workouts for one week. When you begin the next four-week cycle, you'll be at an increased level of fitness, with both a strong immune system and happy hormones to go with it. When you exercise without a plan, you get stale, risk injury, or start taxing your immune system, instead of boosting it.

Women who "exercise" without a PEP usually get frustrated. They don't see the results they expect. More often than not, when you first begin to exercise, you will get results easily. When you reach a foundation of regular exercise, without adding purpose to your activity, however, the pace of your results will slow.

This factor is the one area that most women neglect. They take rest between sets. They do pretty well with a weekly schedule, but this "big" picture is missing. An advantage of a class or a boot camp of six to eight weeks that has a week between sessions is you're gifted this recovery. You're left to exercise on your own between workouts. Few people push themselves as hard alone, as when they work with a trainer, instructor, or the right exercise partner. In this case, a little slacking of your efforts would be ideal. Call it calculated slacking. Although many participants (you could call them type A) often complain, this little break is exactly what helps them gain fitness and avoid injury.

If you're your own personal trainer, build in that same kind of recovery. Every third or fourth week, cut back in the volume of work you do and vary your fitness activities. Don't fall into the trap of doing the same thing over and over again. If you love to run, for instance, you may always turn to running. Or perhaps you work out to the same exercise videos over and over again. During your recovery week, try something else. Previously, it was pointed out that you can't separate your mind and body anymore. You need a mental break from the same type of exercise, as much as you need the physical rest.

If you're used to an exercise class, wipe the cobwebs off your bike and find a bike trail. If you're a runner, accept your friend's offer to take a Zumba class, even if you don't know half the moves. The day will definitely be a recovery day! If you usually strength train on your own, try a group class instead. Try yoga. Don't worry about substituting a cardio workout for a cardio workout or strength for a strength day. Try to get in some of each type of training. The main factor that needs to be considered, in this regard, however, is active recovery. You want cross training, without measuring the outcome of the exercise effort beyond exhibiting a smile or having fun.

ACTIVE VS. PASSIVE RECOVERY

Between intervals, sets, or days after vigorous exercise, choose to engage in active recovery, which is superior to passive recovery. Passive recovery is complete rest, ideally with the cabana boy coming to take your order for green juice (no, not a margarita). Passive recovery can also mean massage, Epsom salt baths, and meditation. On the other hand, active recovery is best. The more you can boost the blood flow to your skeletal muscles, the more good things that will happen to enhance your recovery.

Active recovery is often continuous exercise at a much lower intensity. The intensity of active recovery depends on you. Don't compare yourself to others. Research has found that 30- to 90-minute efforts at 50 percent to 70 percent of $\dot{V}O_2max$ have positive effects on recovery physiology. At that level, you know you're exercising but can go for a long time. Low-intensity exercise like this has been shown to reduce chronic inflammation. More recovery and less work—particularly if you tend to overdo things—could be just the thing that brings you closer to your goals, including unlocking the door to exhibiting your optimal weight. Since inflammation is like road construction in the summer, when you're on your way to a relaxing vacation, reducing it is a priority.

Exercising at a moderate level of intensity for less than 75 minutes has been shown to reduce inflammation and increase levels of positive neurotransmitters, like serotonin and endorphins. Those happy hormones improve brain chemistry. A better brain creates a better body. Long walks outdoors or pedaling along a beautiful bike path, without monitoring your heart rate or shooting for a specific level of intensity, qualify.

In essence, if you don't love to exercise, you don't get a break! Combining passive and active forms of recovery is a simple way to boost your overall recovery, as well as reward you for an active life.

If you plan your exercise efforts wisely, avoiding eccentric types of activities, you'll need less recovery. Eccentric exercises cause more muscle damage and more soreness. Exercises that emphasize eccentric contractions include slow weight training and running, especially downhill. If you swim or cycle on opposite days that you run, for instance, you'll require less recovery time than if you run and lift several days in a row.

Are you overtraining? The more that you experience the following conditions, the greater the chance that you're overtraining and underrecovering:
- Chronic fatigue or feelings of burnout
- Continuous muscle soreness
- Insomnia or sleep disturbances (not present otherwise)

- Consistent elevated resting heart rate (five or more beats per minute)
- Rating of perceived exertion and heart rate at familiar exercise intensities drifting higher or lower
- High number of competitions or races
- A significant increase in exercise intensity
- A significant increase in exercise volume
- An increase in the level of exposure to environmental stressors
- Changes in family, friendships, or social relationships
- New job demands
- Loss of lean muscle weight
- Changes in diet or a loss of appetite
- An increase in depression, anxiety, anger, tension, forgetfulness
- A decrease in joy, sense of humor, or enjoyment of normally pleasurable activities

Resolve personal conflicts, improve your diet, and take a recovery break from your regular exercise routine to relieve symptoms of overtraining, or overstressing. You'll allow your concentration of hormones to return to a functional level. Both too little and too much exercise can get between you and your ability to look and feel great.

HOW DO YOU KNOW IF YOU'RE RECOVERED?

Baseline measurements are critical for assessing how well your recovery training sessions are progressing. There are a couple ways to measure the level of success of such recovery bouts.

Simply taking your resting heart rate (RHR) before you start training gives you one indicator for comparison. Record your heart rates during workouts and how quickly you recover from intervals. When these heart rates or times are "off" consistently, you'll know you're in your personal "overdoing it" range and need to adjust.

An elevated resting heart rate of 5 to 10 beats or more per minute three days in a row or a slower than normal recovery are indications that you're overtraining and that another rest day is warranted. By the time you notice a spike in your RHR, you've been overtraining for a while. Use the 30-day tracking chart in Appendix A-6 to monitor your status. Then, you can adjust your training schedule, based on your findings. If your resting heart rate suddenly increases for a few days, follow with a few light days of recovery.

There's a new method of checking recovery that may become more common in the future. Monitors that measure heart rate variability (HRV) get feedback directly from your nervous system. The nervous system is highly in tune with stress. Knowing what's going on can tell you whether your overall level of stress (and cortisol) requires adjustments in your exercise routine or whether you're ready for more of the same.

HRV represents shifts in the time between heartbeats. You're going to get intimate with your heart rate. It's not just your heart rate during and after exercise anymore. You want to know how much time between heartbeats. Nosy!

For example, say that your resting heart rate is 60 beats per minute. Well, 60 beats per minute should represent a heart beating in one-second intervals, but that is not what actually happens. For example, the heart can beat at the 0.8, 1.2, 1.3 or 0.7 marks to produce a 60-bpm average. Researchers have found that increased HRV is normal and more desirable than that predictable one-second interval (based on a heart rate of 60 beats per minute).

A heart rate with a lot of variability between beats means that your system is working to reduce stressors and keep you running smoothly. On the other hand, a low HRV means that your body is still under a lot of stress. Go figure. It's a little like when life is chaotic, and you have a sudden need to organize the spice rack or to vacuum. Too much order is not always good.

High variability in heart rate means that you can handle a challenging exercise session. Low variability means that you've got too much stress response already and cannot readily handle more. You won't get results you want if you work out hard, when you're not recovered.

HRV monitors are fairly inexpensive and work with a heart-rate chest band. A daily reading takes less than five minutes. To understand how your system is dealing with stressors and what type of exercise intensity is best, use a HRV. A fitness professional working with you on this can help interpret your HRV results and adjust your exercise programming.

Measuring hormone levels is not always feasible, convenient, or even completely accurate. Heart rate variability, on the other hand, is direct feedback to your inner stressor or calm. The beauty of direct and specialized feedback like HRV is that it can provide custom feedback relative to everything that affects you, including exercise, diet, sleep, age, gender, and stressors.

On a simpler level, observe changes in your day-to-day activity and mood for clues about your recovery status. Your sleep can suffer if you're overexercising or just overloaded with stressors. Remember that a body that's already stressed may not respond well to vigorous exercise. That's not the message you've been sent either from the media or from fitness marketers who want you to register for boot camp. You suddenly may not be able to fall asleep or stay asleep, when that's not typically a problem. Don't just assume it's due to manic menopause. If you're irritable, moody, or feel depressed, back off exercising and see if that helps you.

At this point, you've read about how balancing your exercise intensity and volume, with rest between sets, between same-day workouts, or over weeks and months, is an integral part of recovery. The little voice inside your head that might be telling you that you don't need recovery because you're tough and you're not tired needs to stifle it. Optimal fitness, weight loss, and energy will not happen without recovery.

MORE WAYS TO FACILITATE RECOVERY

A number of methods of non-exercise rest and recovery exist. Some are active, and some are passive, including the following:

- Nutrition
- Stretching
- Foam rolling
- Massage
- Compression
- Sleep
- Hydrotherapy
- Life stress reduction

PASSIVE RECOVERY: NUTRITION

When you realize that everything you eat and that every exercise, bedtime, and stress-handling choice is either sending a message to your body to burn fat and build muscle or to store fat, you'll start to make choices for your best health.

Chapter 3 addressed another R&R—remove and reintroduce. The body needs recovery from dieting. It also may need to recover and heal from inflammation in the gut caused by dieting, from taking medicine, or from experiencing stress.

Clearly, refueling for recovery is complicated by the fact that you may be trying to lose or maintain weight. Over 50 percent of women (including those over 50) who exercise state that weight loss is their primary reason for moving. If you resort to dieting in an effort to boost weight loss, you slow your recovery. Calorie reduction can become an additional stressor on bodily systems that can end up decreasing exercise performance, disrupting hormone response to nutrition, and slowing your metabolism.

Super strenuous workouts create the inflammation known as acidosis, which corrodes muscles. Bye-bye muscle means hello fat. Adjusting your nutrition will help balance your body's internal pH and reduce its level of acidosis inflammation. Alkaline foods reduce inflammation, while more acidic foods like dairy and animal-based foods increase inflammation. Drink lemon-infused water. Focus on plant-based foods and berries.

The consumption of more vegetables, fruits, and foods rich in omega 3 fats to reduce inflammation is important to exercisers who are altering their internal physiology every day. They can also be beneficial to you, even if you're only exercising moderately for good health. Poor nutrition can compromise your ability to get what you want.

Right after a tough workout, a protein and carbohydrate combination within 30 minutes of finishing helps you begin the recovery and repair of your muscles. Chocolate milk meets the recommended ratio of 1:4 proteins to carbohydrates. For adults over 50, there is evidence that protein before or after a particularly hard cardio or a resistance training workout will help stop catabolism, the breakdown of your sexy toned muscles. Eating either a high-quality protein-rich (i.e., 25 to 30 grams) meal within 90 minutes post-exercise or taking in 24 to 40 grams of protein with a protein drink, if a meal is not planned soon, will help you keep the muscle and lose the fat.

Consuming post-exercise protein is especially important if it's been several hours since your last meal when you exercise. If you have performed light or moderate exercise, and you're eating an adequate amount of calories and protein, you may not need to include a pre- or post-exercise snack.

Exercising "too much" is not statistically the problem in America. On the other hand, many women go through cycles of overdoing and underdoing. If you're eating well, sleeping well, and exercising daily, but can't make the scale or your belt loop budge, you may actually be doing too much exercise, as well as achieving too little recovery.

The Mediterranean diet is favored for reducing oxidative stress and boosting recovery. Oxidative stress is an imbalance between the production of free radicals and the ability of the body to counteract or detoxify their harmful effects through neutralization by antioxidants. The two qualities of the Mediterranean diet that boost antioxidants are high levels of healthy omega 3 fats from fish (low mercury options) and the prevalence of non-starchy green leafy vegetables. Because skeletal muscles use the most oxygen, damage there is eminent. In reality, loss of your lean muscle is the last thing you want to happen after you commit to exercise. The high-quality protein from this diet also boosts recovery.

ACTIVE RECOVERY: STRETCHING AND FOAM ROLLING

While static stretching of the muscles should be done after exercise, it *can* also be done before. Ideally, you'll combine those long-holding stretches with another technique that targets your fascia—or connective tissue. *Dynamic stretching* is another part of effective stretching that can enhance your flexibility. Keep in mind that even when you're "tight," it doesn't always mean you need to stretch.

Your connective tissue is something that rarely comes up if you're talking about weight loss, but it should. The condition of your connective tissue depends on your age and what you've done to keep your tissue healthy, hydrated, and flexible. You can't do a thing about your age or the past, but you can start feeling better today with a technique called self-myofascial release (SMR).

SMR combines pressure and movement. While not as enjoyable as a massage therapist kneading you, SMR is convenient, economical, and available on-call.

SMR techniques help release the tissue below the skin. As you age, your tissue becomes less resilient. If you've been ignoring your tissue, it's all bound up instead of nicely aligned and springy. You're about to explore a new way to rock and roll. You're going to take your rock and roll it.

You want to use a soft foam roller or ball and apply less pressure when you begin. Use a tool with a large surface area, as opposed to small. Think of a squishy foam roller as a friend, and a golf ball as a foe.

Your "more is better" thinking should end at this point. Goldilocks' pressure is best: not too much, not too little, but just right. Your muscles should remain pliable, and your movements should be slow and controlled. You defeat the inherent purpose of SMR, if you apply so much pressure that it hurts. No pain, no brain.

If you can persuade a partner or feed quarters to a child, they can do this rolling for you either with a rolling pin (seriously, were you using it anyway?) or with more flexible tools on the market that have been specifically designed for this purpose. (Refer to Appendix B-5 for information on the "stick.")

Fascia is made up of 70 to 80 percent water. Dehydration of your fascia can be the cause of pain fatigue, bloating, headaches, and muscle aches. Did you see bloating in there? Time to roll.

Studies show that foam rolling (SMR) prior to static stretching increases flexibility better than stretching alone, SMR alone, or skipping that cool-down altogether (gasp). Another study found that dynamic stretching—the type most often recommended in warm-ups or flowing yoga—can be a very effective addition to your exercise routine.

You can improve the flexibility and hydration of your fascia at any age. Make the trilogy of SMR, dynamic stretching, and static stretching a part of your regular routine. One or two times a week, for a few minutes at a time, is all it takes to generate lasting cumulative effects. More isn't better. Your connective tissue needs time to synthesize after you roll. Once it does, you'll move with more freedom, while your program may not be satisfying from a standpoint of immediate gratification, since your progress will be slow over the first weeks, consistent regular foam roller and stretching training will get lasting results within 6 to 24 months. Part #2 of your three-part trilogy follows.

Dynamic movement primes your flexibility pump. Actively engaging targeted muscles in movement before a stretch can increase the effectiveness of your stretch. If you've done Pilates or yoga, you may identify similar patterns of dynamic flow, followed by held poses or exercise sequences. Both are credited with improving mobility and function. If your personal discipline goddess has vacated, try a class or DVD to help keep you accountable until you're hooked, because of how good it feels. As such, your after 50 flexibility formula should include the following elements:

- SMR
- Dynamic movement
- Stretching

SMR

A quick introduction to self-myofascial release, beginning with your hands and feet, involves the following steps. Use a soft ball, like a racquet or tennis ball. This type of SMR can help with your grip, provide arthritis relief, and introduce you to the concept of SMR, before you have to juggle your body weight and your positioning on the floor, using a foam roller.

❏ Hand Release

This exercise addresses arthritis pain in the fingers and wrist.

Part #1:
- Place your right hand, with your palm down, on a malleable ball, supported on a table.
- Press your hand onto the ball; you can use your left hand to increase the level of pressure.
- Lift and splay your fingers and hold for four seconds, and then gently close your fingers around the ball.
- Repeat four times.

Part #2:
- Gently roll the ball across the top of your right hand, with your fingers splayed, from your wrist and over and between each finger.
- Repeat the sequence on your left hand.
- Follow with a straight-arm wrist extension, flexion, and rotation. With your arm extended, put your palm up like a stop sign. Then, point your fingers down and circle your wrist around several times, both clockwise and counterclockwise.

❏ Foot Release

This exercise addresses ankle range of motion, plantar fasciitis, and foot pain.

Part #1:
- Roll the arch of your right foot across the ball, from front to back.
- Repeat four times, from your medial to your lateral arch.
- Lean your arms and torso across your thigh to increase the level of pressure.
- Repeat with your left foot.

Part #2:
- Place the ball behind your toes, under the ball of your right foot.
- Press and curl your toes down and around the ball; hold for four seconds.
- Press again, while lifting your toes up and out; hold for four seconds.
- Repeat four times.

- Follow with plantar flexion and dorsiflexion.
- Repeat with your left foot.

PASSIVE RECOVERY

Passive recovery, discussed earlier in this chapter, involves complete rest from exercise. Though not as effective as active recovery at enhancing recovery by stimulating blood flow to skeletal muscles, passive recovery has its benefits. For example, passive recovery can decrease the level of the hormones that interfere with recovery, as well as increase the level of those hormones that can have a positive impact on recovery, or both. Examples of proven passive recovery methods include the following:

❑ Passive Recovery: Massage

Massage has been well documented for its potential to reduce inflammation and reduce cortisol. Touch may boost oxytocin and serotonin. In turn, it may enhance sleep. What more do you need to know other than it feels good?

Athletes have used massage for years to enhance their recovery. Because there are several variations to choose from, you should ask a professional before you're under the sheet. Be sure that whatever massage therapist you select will adjust to your pressure and your needs. Some people enjoy a massage as often as once a week, while others take a massage on a monthly basis. While people who wait until they need it may enjoy the massage, they will not enjoy their life between massages as much.

❑ Passive Recovery: Compression

Massage is one form of muscle compression. The goal of compression is enhanced circulation. At the present time, there are several methods of compression used by both athletes and non-athletes. For example, compression garments, which can be worn before, during, or after exercise, may help recovery. They help improve circulation, as well as help prevent blood pooling or fluid retention. You can buy compression tights or shirts or use muscle-targeted sleeves designed for calves, thighs, and arms. While individual results vary, there have been few, if any, negative side effects reported from their use.

Compression boots are like sleeves you slip into that fill with air. You can invest in them yourself or use them at health clubs that cater to athletes or competitive age-group athletes.

❑ Passive Recovery: Sleep

Sleep is the ultimate form of rest. Read more about how and why to get adequate sleep, as well as how to establish your personal sleep needs in Chapter 5. It is during the deepest phase of sleep that your body most regenerates. If you're tempted to cut into sleep to rise early or stay up late, imagine that you're having a slice of rich chocolate cake, with two-inch thick frosting, and it is going right to your hips where it plans to take up residence.

❏ Passive Recovery: Hydrotherapy

While warm baths by themselves are relaxing, Epsom salt soaks can reduce muscle cramps and further enhance relaxation. Magnesium is known as a natural stress reliever. It calms your level of anxiety, which serves as an aid for preventing insomnia. If you soak with two cups of Epsom salts in a standard tub, two or three times a week, your body will absorb magnesium through the skin, if you're deficient in this particular mineral. It's an alternative to taking magnesium supplements. By the same token, it won't harm you, if you're already consuming enough.

In (literal) contrast to the relaxing effect of a warm bath are contrast baths of cold (55-degrees Fahrenheit) and warm (105-degrees Fahrenheit) water. Immerging or placing a sore part of your body in each bath for four to six minutes and then alternating two or three times between the two can decrease swelling and inflammation. This sequence can be intense. If you do choose to undergo such punishment, use your tub for the ice bath and a warm shower or a Jacuzzi can suffice for the warm bath if you don't have two tubs.

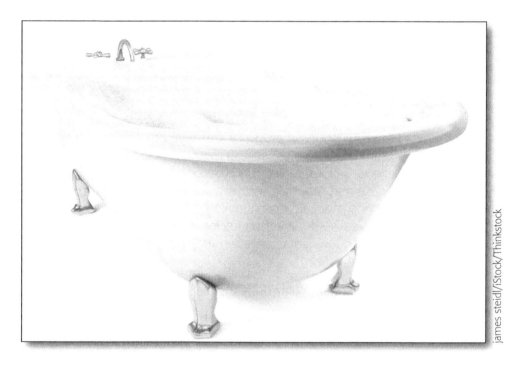

james steidl/iStock/Thinkstock

Reduce your easy swimming to a more relaxed chill effort. Even floating in water has been suggested to help increase the blood-pumping mechanism of your body that is needed for clearing toxins from your system.

❑ Passive Recovery: Life Stress Reduction

Stop stressing. As elusive as this last tip may seem, it can be one of the most effective secrets of improving your fitness results. Proper use of exercise to improve stress levels is fine. Throughout this book, you'll read that you don't want to address the symptoms you're facing. You want to fix the problem. Addressing the source of your stressors will help you eliminate a negative hormone cascade that accompanies them. When you can do that, your exercise prescription for optimal health will become far easier to manage. Don't run from your stress. Address it. Then run (or Zumba or swim, etc.) for joy.

Turn to Appendix A-11 and complete the Stress Toolbox Worksheet. Then, start tracking activities that boost your recovery, remove toxins, and provide feedback from your body about what it needs with the 30-Day After 50 Fitness Tracker (Appendix A-6).

FEATURED EXPERT

Joe Friel

❑ How to Recover

As strange as it may seem, training as if you are trying to become overtrained is necessary for high performance in sport, regardless of your age. You can't get to where you want to go by taking it easy. The process of becoming fit requires that you do workouts that stress your body to a level for which it is not currently adapted.

Subsequently, you will become tired, which will upset the body. As a result, your body manages the situation by adapting and becoming "stronger." You can't do such a workout only one time and expect to reap great benefits, however. A high level of fitness requires that you engage in your workouts repeatedly for some period of time, over and over for several days or for a couple of weeks. The key to doing this successfully is building in recovery days, when you back off between your hard sessions, to let your body catch up. It's during rest and recovery that the body adapts.

In this regard, the key issue is what is a stressful workout? Essentially, a stressful workout is a hard workout, one that is either longer than you generally do, highly intense, or both. Typically, such a session should require around 48 to 72 hours between workouts in order to recover before doing the next hard one. During those two or three days, you should wither perform an easy, active-recovery workout or rest completely. Most over-50 athletes can generally manage two or three such hard sessions in a week, with active recovery or rest days between them.

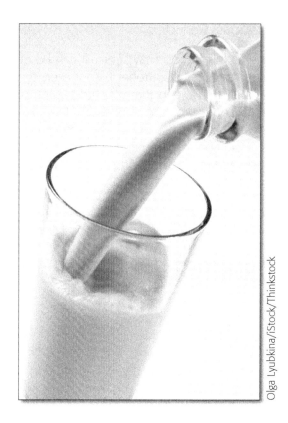

Quick recovery after a hard workout is one of the keys to success in endurance sports. The sooner you are recovered, the sooner you can do another such workout. The more hard workouts you can do in a given period of time, the more fit you become. The more fit you are, the faster you race. In other words, the key is to recover quickly.

What can you do to recover quickly after a hard session? The following is what I tell the athletes I coach to do and in the order they should do them. Not everyone can do each of the following steps after every hard workout, because things like a career and other responsibilities that demand your time may get in the way. Just do the best job you can, realizing that on some days, it will be easier to plug in more of these six suggested steps than on other days:

• Athletes who eat a high-carbohydrate diet should take in carbs within 30 minutes of finishing a hard workout. Most individuals prefer this in a liquid form. It could be fruit juice, chocolate milk, a blender homebrew you make, or a commercial recovery drink—something you like the taste of. Depending on body size, your experience, and how hard the workout was, you'll probably need between 200 and 400 calories. You'll know when you've had enough. Don't take in more than what feels comfortable. According to the latest recovery research, it may also be a good idea to include some protein, either as a powder added to your drink or from real food (which is preferable). About 10 grams (40 calories) is probably adequate. This protein and these carbs don't have to be expensive, exotic, or designed by a "scientist." If you eat a high-fat diet, instead of a high-carb one, just be sure to have your typical snack after the workout, such as nuts, nut butter, cheese, avocado, coconut milk, or whatever you like. Again, include some protein in your snack, such as a boiled egg or a tuna salad.

- As soon as possible after the workout, elevate your legs. For example, lay on the floor with your feet and legs on a chair or against the wall. This positioning will take the load off of your heart and encourage the redistribution of fluids that have pooled in your legs. A few minutes of doing this is usually enough.

- Take a nap. This suggestion is one that most people can't seem to fit into their schedule. Young pro athletes seem to nap regularly. On the other hand, they don't usually have to rush off to work or to some other appointment. It's during sleep that the body adapts as anabolic (rebuilding) hormones are subsequently released. Thirty to sixty minutes is probably enough to help speed recovery.

- Drink fluids to completely satisfy thirst the remainder of the day (there is no "schedule" or precise amount you must drink). Water is the number one choice. Sports drinks are okay immediately post-workout, but as the day wears on, these drinks increasingly become poor choices for fluids. Your cells don't need to be saturated with sugar, sodium, and other "stuff" for the remainder of the day.

- Again, if you eat a high-carb diet, in your first "real" meal after a hard workout, include some dietary starch. The best options in this instance are potatoes, sweet potatoes, and yams. It may also be appropriate to eat some grains (bread, bagels, cereal, corn, rice, etc.). Some individuals prefer vegetables to grains at this time, since veggies are richer in micronutrients than are grains. After that meal, return to eating primarily veggies, fruits, and protein, while reducing your intake of starches, because, as was previously noted, starches are less rich in vitamins and minerals. The primary concern at this time is long-range recovery. Micronutrients are needed for that. If you've done a good job of taking in sugar immediately post-workout and adequate starch in the first post-workout meal, then you shouldn't need any more starch or sugar again for the remainder of the day. If you eat a high-fat diet, instead of a high-carb one, eat what you normally have for meals the remainder of the day.

- The most important form of recovery comes in sleep the night immediately after your hard session. As was noted previously, this period is when adaptation takes place, and you actually become more fit. A full night of sleep is the key. In other words, it's best to sleep until you awake naturally— not to an alarm clock. That often means going to bed early. Again, a lot of people simply can't fit an early bedtime into their lifestyles, due to so many other commitments. On the other hand, it is important to realize that this is the recovery method that will give you the greatest return on investment.

While the aforementioned is what I have advised those individuals I've coached to do in order to recover quickly from a stressful workout, we often wind up modifying things to better fit their unique situations. These changes frequently involve the time of day they do certain types of workouts. For example, when doing two sessions in a day, their workouts may need to be arranged so that the one that will be more convenient to recover after, in terms of meals, sleep, and rest, is the harder one.

Joe Friel is the author of 15 books on training for endurance sports. His latest is Fast After 50. *He can be reached through his blog at joefrielsblog.com.*

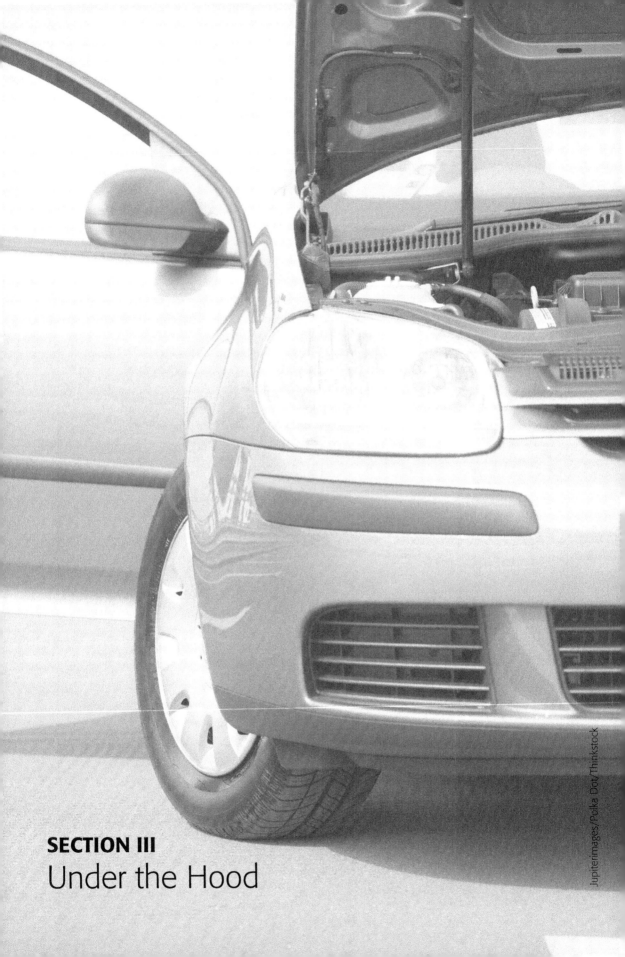

SECTION III
Under the Hood

Jupiterimages/Polka Dot/Thinkstock

If you're in hormone hell, keep going.

CHAPTER 8

Hormone Hell to Hormone Heal

You bought the gloves for the weight room. You purchased some of those lulu knock-offs at Target. *Damn*, admit it, you look the part. You changed your diet, and now, you not only *think* you're eating right, you *are*. Still, though, no change. From the shoulders up, you feel young. You want to throw caution to the wind, go crazy and topless (the car), but first muffin-topless, with or without the wind blowing in your hair sounds amazing.

If you are in hormone hell, no amount of exercise or cutting calories is going to make you skinny. In fact, every effort you're making could be pushing your vision of being a goddess further away. Sleep won't leave you feeling rested, and your usual sources of pleasure won't be much source of joy. In this non-intuitive chapter, you're going to find out that women are blessed. You've been gifted with far more unpredictable hormones and phases of life than you ever asked for.

When is it time to test? Should you even invest in a test? What if you test normal, and you still feel lousy? We're going to address all of these issues and walk through the hormone minefield—one by one.

Your brain is hormone central. The hypothalamus and pituitary gland in the brain control how much hormone is released from the various glands. When you feel stressed, that's a sign your brain is pumping out stress hormones. If sustained over months and years, that situation can ruin your health and make you a nervous wreck. Even temporarily though, it can prevent what used to work for you from helping you shape up and lose those extra pounds. Women used to call that seasonal weight cycling winter weight. If you're talking about it in June and have to ask which winter, it's time for change.

This story unfolds, as estrogen gets your attention. For women approaching 50 and beyond, estrogen is the squeaky wheel. Around menopause, even if going through it was no big deal, the change in sex hormones (more on them later) causes a shift. For example, you experience weight accumulation around the middle or some of your body parts start moving downtown. You may weigh the same, but you're not the same proportion or tone. What really starts causing all the problems though is something else. Enter cortisol.

CORTISOL

Meet cortisol, otherwise known as the stress hormone. Your brain has the ability to selectively activate the fight, flight, or defeat responses. This activation occurs every time you perceive your hassles as either a challenge to control or a loss of control. Each option uniquely affects your body functions.

The "fight" or "flight" stress responses cause your heart to beat faster and harder, as well as release more free fatty acids into the blood. Picture a sudden emergency at school or work for one of your loved ones or having to finish a report in a flurry to beat a deadline.

The "defeat" stress response leads to enhanced fat *creation* (lipogenesis), visceral obesity (deep belly fat), breakdown of tissues, and suppression of the immune system. Picture yourself in a dead-end job, feeling hopeless without a light at the end of the tunnel.

Cortisol is somewhat of a hormone superhero. If it weren't so obnoxious, you would be impressed. It can move fat from storage depots and relocate it to fat-cell deposits deep in the belly. This scenario is not desirable. Cortisol also helps baby fat cells to grow up into mature fat cells, which is also not desirable. Finally, cortisol may act as an anti-inflammatory agent, suppressing your immune system during times of physical and psychological stress. Three strikes you're out.

Hypothetically, say that you're in a high stress job, and you start a diet and begin exercising more often. You may notice that you start getting more colds. Your system just can't handle it all. All of this can stimulate you to want food that is high in carbs, fat, and/or sugar. Cortisol indirectly influences your appetite by regulating other chemicals that are released during stress. She's a bad-girl ringleader.

Cortisol is like a gatekeeper to regulate how cells function and how other hormones get used. If your adrenal glands aren't functioning because there is *too little* cortisol present, the response—weight gain and lethargy—mimics low thyroid function, even though the gland is working properly. You read that right. Cortisol being too low is a problem too. You really want to find the sweet spot. This factor will be a theme. Finding your right balance is the object of this game.

This amazing body you live in works in integration, not isolation. So, you either have the social mixer of the year going on, or you have cliques, and no one is talking.

❑ Small Amounts of Cortisol Save Your Life; Large Amounts of Cortisol Kill You

Too much stress over a period of time, combined with poor coping habits, even the way you think about stress, may cause physical, chemical, and hormonal imbalances in your body, leading to disease and death if left unchecked.

You have 400 percent more cortisol receptors and greater blood flow in your visceral (belly) fat than in your subcutaneous (pinchable) fat. On top of that, there is a resourceful little enzyme there that can make its own cortisol in belly fat, which compounds your expanding elastic waistband problem. The more weight you have to lose, the more this enzyme is expressed. The end result is that cortisol helps you accumulate fat and enlarge the fat cells already in the belly. Some kind of help you can do without.

If cortisol were at the junior high dance, cortisol would be the one spiking the punch and stepping on toes. No one wants to dance with cortisol. Ah, but," Principal Stress" comes in and insists.

Cortisol obviously directly affects fat storage and weight gain when you're stressed. As if it's not bad enough that you could die from at least 80 stress-causing diseases thanks to cortisol, before you die, you get fat.

In addition to higher stress levels, lack of sleep is also associated with an increase in cortisol. An increase in cortisol is related to sugar cravings. Sugar consumption leads to insulin release, which results in fat metabolism coming to a halt. You already guessed that extra sugar is not what you need to lose weight. In fact, sugar has a much greater impact on fat and obesity than eating fat.

There's a natural dip in cortisol between three and four o'clock in the afternoon. If you really crash or are tempted to break into the vending machine, eat a snack between two and three o'clock to offset the cortisol low that's coming.

Any stressors that your mind and body have to deal with contribute to your increasing potential to gain and decreasing ability to lose weight. Remember that cortisol has some redeeming qualities. It can be either good or bad for fat storage. The net impact of cortisol depends on how much and how long it's high or low in your body, and what else is going on with you at the moment.

Many types of aerobic and anaerobic exercise have been shown to be effective interventions in reducing or managing stress. Choosing the right type and dose of exercise to help balance your cortisol levels is key. When you're uber-stressed, yoga may be a better fat-burning friend than an hour of a high-intensity boot camp. As you will learn, a calorie is not a calorie. This factor is true both when you eat and when you exercise.

Consider the relationship between cortisol and growth hormone (GH) when you choose an exercise. (You'll read about GH shortly.) Either a challenging exercise of a short duration or a soothing, leisurely nature walk creates optimal balance between the two hormones. A little cortisol is good, a lot is bad. Optimal growth hormone helps you maintain lean muscle tissue. Too much exercise when you're overstressed can increase cortisol and decrease growth hormone to the degree exercise actually backfires on you.

You can eat to support cortisol. Cortisol's natural rhythm follows our own—or it should. It naturally peaks in the morning around eight and rises and falls during the day, as needed, reaching its lowest level while we're sleeping.

So, naturally, you'd think eating your heartier meals early in the day and eating smaller lighter meals at night would help keep the weight off and hormones in balance. This point is where it gets complicated.

The opposite can be true. If, for example, you're having a lot of trouble sleeping and experiencing cravings and energy crash, the rules change. A form of carb-cycling, i.e., shifting some of your intake of high-quality carb sources to later in the day, can offset low cortisol levels that make you edgy or anxious or crave something, other than carrots and hummus. While skewing some carb intake to later in the day is counterintuitive, it can improve your sleep and reset your circadian clock.

While the aforementioned might take some getting used to, think of your unbalanced hormones as having the flu. Spinach is uber-healthy. You wouldn't have a spinach salad with the stomach flu, though, right? So, for your "sick" hormones, we have a different "best" plan. Once things do balance again, you'll be back to the norm, but ignoring your "flu-like" symptoms won't help you heal your hormones.

If your stress cravings seem higher late day, fatigue is a big problem, or sweet dreams are elusive, *then* include healthy complex carbs at night. Invite a sweet potato or brown rice to dinner. Furthermore, *if* you're sleeping poorly, *then* adjust your exercise regimen, so that your late day activity is yoga or an easy stroll.

You're going to hear more about cortisol and its influence on other hormones. When cortisol teams up with insulin, for instance, you're up against two belly-fat bullies.

INSULIN

Insulin comes to the party when you eat and your blood sugar rises. After a particularly high carbohydrate meal or a sugar donut, you can bet insulin is knocking at your door. Even fruit, with all its nutrients, is sugar. Once insulin is present, fat metabolism comes to a halt. At that point, any excess calories are more likely to be stored as fat.

What's worse, if insulin is present in your body, it's less likely that fat will be burned, *even if* there is a calorie deficit. And, you thought cortisol was bad. Well, it is. Cortisol is basically your two-faced backstabbing you-know-what.

A little cortisol for a short time, as in times of stress or when you're engaged in a short bout of high-intensity exercise, helps you burn fat. In the presence of insulin, though, fat-burning is blunted.

When you eat sugar or foods easily converted to sugar, insulin is released. A devastating situation for your fat-fighting agenda would be to drink either a glass (or half bottle) of wine late in the afternoon on an empty stomach or a big glass of orange juice first thing in the morning, chased down by a bowl of stars and moons cereal.

The goal is to avoid spikes in blood sugar. Stabilize your blood sugar, and you reduce the release of insulin. Decrease your intake of sweets and starches, and get regular exercise. Exercise will also help you with your production of growth hormone, which is important for the results you want.

GROWTH HORMONE

What could be better than decreasing belly-fat deposits and enhancing lean, toned muscle while you sleep? Growth hormone (GH) is responsible for both, and the majority of growth hormone is released while you sleep. Remember that cortisol levels go up when sleep is down. In other words, before you dash out to the running shoe store, you might want to stop at the mattress store.

Your production of GH decreases with age, which is unfortunate, since it helps burn fat and boosts muscle recovery so that you can gain and keep lean muscle. Along with cortisol, GH helps determine how much fat is deposited in your belly.

You can't change your age, but improving your sleep hygiene and exercising right can enhance GH production. First, you should pillow talk.

In normal healthy people, the major period of GH release is in the first period of stage three sleep during the night. You go through stage three about seven times during a good night's sleep. You have five stages of sleep altogether. Stages three and four are the most important for human growth hormone. Stage three is the beginning of deep sleep.

Because GH is released in stages three and four, some fitness and sports performance trainers call sleep "the athlete's steroid." GH helps maintain and repair muscles and cells. As such, it's the key to improving athletic performance. It's your drug of choice to improve your superhero middle-aged ability to rule the world and rock the skinny jeans.

As we age, most of us spend less time in deep sleep. As such, our secretion of GH decreases. With lower than normal levels of GH, the body can't properly control the proportion of fat to muscle. When this situation happens, we tend to store more fat in the belly. Accordingly, besides working on ways to enhance your sleep (snooze to lose by reading Chapter 5), you can exercise to optimize GH.

A number of studies suggest that exercise-induced GH release is best achieved with exercise undertaken at or just above your lactate threshold. That exercise intensity is the one at which lactic acid—the burn—accumulates in the blood. What's that feel like? You're breathless. You're really working. What's the good news? When this exercise is done right, you just do it for a short time. Hit it and quit it. (Really, it's HIIT it and quit it: high intensity interval training; read more about this topic in Chapter 4.)

Exercise training above the lactate threshold appears to amplify GH release, even at rest, for at least 24 hours. Now, you're talking. This factor is why HIIT and a good dose of strength training can be so beneficial for you. It's also why other types of exercise may backfire.

To eat in a way that supports GH function, you should focus on quality protein and avoid high-glycemic load carbohydrates. In other words, reduce your intake of most starchy veggies and pastas, fruits, and sugary snacks. Insulin and cortisol levels will both benefit from the same advice.

All of the aforementioned makes GH seem like a big help in the battle of bat wings and belly fat. There's a downside to GH, however—the synthetic type of GH that is often given to dairy cows, so they get fat and produce more milk. If you're drinking dairy milk or milk products containing those hormones, essentially *you're taking them* too and—bingo—if they do what they're intended to do so well for cows, they're contributing to your weight gain. Kick your intake of dairy for a week and see what happens. Then, if/when you reintroduce it, go for the organic labels that indicate that the dairy was produced hormone-free.

ADRENALINE

Your adrenal glands moderate your stress response, as well as regulate other hormones. Cortisol is one adrenal-regulated hormone. Remember cortisol? Too high or too low, it's a naughty girl. It's a broken record, but balance is your best friend.

If your adrenal glands continue to produce cortisol for long periods of time, eventually they have a decreased level of ability to do it. Instead, they produce adrenaline. Adrenaline makes you feel irritable, shaky, lightheaded, and anxious. Been there?

When adrenal dysfunction is healed, a lot of problems can be relieved. Sometimes, though, adrenal dysfunction is misinterpreted as a thyroid problem. When your adrenals are overworking and high, the natural response in your body *is* low thyroid. It's saying, well if you're going to do this, I'll do that. It's quite an amazing way that the body is trying to stay in balance, somehow.

Your problem comes if your low thyroid is just a symptom. Ideally, you wouldn't treat the thyroid first. Focus on what's causing that symptom. Manage your stressors. Look closely at whether you're trying to play superwoman.

You need to ask, even if no one else does, *how is my stress level? How close is my daily schedule to my ideal? How is my diet?* Without a close look at what might be causing the problem, your treatment efforts could easily be targeted at the *symptoms*, not the root, of your problem.

Your first natural line of defense is lifestyle habits. *If* you decrease your level of stress (i.e., adjust your emotional *response* to stressors and change what, when, and how you eat), *then* you may be able to reverse your adrenal fatigue. Shifting the time and type of exercise you do is also stress-smart. Exercise with more intensity should come in the morning. For afternoon and evening exercise, you should think "light at night." Practice yoga or take a walk outdoors after dinner. When you have to make an adjustment in your life, based on a commute or work schedule, it's worth asking if you can manipulate your schedule with an hour later start at work. If your system is really broken, it's worth asking if you should find another job or move closer to work.

If you resist eating breakfast because you're not hungry, it might be a symptom of having a decreased liver function, which is a sign of adrenal fatigue. Accordingly, increasing your intake of fiber to a level above the normal recommended level (21 grams a day for women over 50) could help reduce the recirculation of fat and toxins from the gut back to the liver.

If your liver is dysfunctional, it will not manufacture adequate amounts of the good cholesterol (HDL), which travels out of the liver to scavenge the unhealthy cholesterol (LDL) from the blood vessel walls. That said, testing high for cholesterol could be a clue, rather than the primary problem. Work with your physician on righting your diet and reduce your toxic load (refer to Chapter 6) to see if you can change what's happening naturally.

Your adrenal glands (as well as your thyroid) need iodine in order for them to work properly. If you're iodine deficient and other substances that *are* present in your body are mistaken for iodine, they won't produce the same result. Your body can get confused. The wrong substances intercept the ball and run the wrong way. This problem of mistaken identity is real. Your system can go haywire because of it. Hypothyroid patients are advised to avoid toothpaste with fluoride, and drink purified water free of fluoride and chlorine, since these two compounds can be used for the wrong job.

If you eat seafood, sea vegetables, eggs, and dairy regularly, chances are your diet is high enough in iodine, but it is worth checking with your physician. Don't just self-supplement with iodine, since it can be toxic at too high levels.

It's not hard to figure out how the adrenal glands can get overworked. The female hormone estrogen is actually produced from testosterone. Women require adequate amounts of testosterone to feel strong, energetic, and sexy. If you find your way back to sexy, your other hormones will benefit too. Around menopause, when the ovaries no longer produce adequate amounts of sex hormones, the adrenal glands take over the role of the ovaries to a significant degree.

The aforementioned factor is like you losing your executive assistant at work and picking up her responsibilities on top of yours. At that point, your adrenal production of sex hormones becomes much more important. If you have healthy adrenal glands, you will be the most likely to feel good and have fewer symptoms during menopause. This factor helps to explain why feelings of adrenal fatigue are also most likely to show up at this point.

❑ *Signs and Symptoms of Adrenal Fatigue:*

- *Caffeine is a must to get up; sugar or more caffeine is also mandatory during the day.*
- *Tiredness, sleepiness, grogginess during the day*
- *Difficulty sleeping, even if exhausted (wired and tired)*
- *Salt and sweet cravings*
- *Loss of body hair*
- *Lack of sexual desires*
- *Low blood pressure*
- *Abrupt weight loss or weight gain*
- *Trouble recuperating from illness*

❑ *Causes of Adrenal Fatigue:*

- *Emotions: fear, worry, a lack of pleasurable experiences*
- *Circumstances that cause helplessness: prolonged financial hardship, negative personal relationships*
- *Physical stressors: too much to do, a lack of rest and recovery, poor diet, chronic illness or pain, excessive exercise, environmental toxins*

The reality is it may not be a big dramatic event that triggers adrenal fatigue. It may be from ignoring your symptoms for too long and just doing what a woman does. You exhibit a get-her-done-at all-costs attitude. Usually yours. When you get to the point where you notice the hormone account is low, you're probably really bottoming out.

If you're over 50, under stress, have compromised your diet, or overexercised in an effort to lose weight, there's a good chance that your adrenals need to heal. If adrenal fatigue symptoms resonate with you, then reduce those physical stressors by learning to delegate or ditch. Reduce toxin exposure, and consider whether your health is worth the situation you're tolerating.

The adrenal glands are very fatty organs and to function efficiently, they must receive adequate amounts of healthy fats. If your mindset is "fat makes you fat," start trying to lose *those* six inches of stinking-thinking between your ears.

THYROID

Thyroid problems are very common in women around the time that they experience menopause. As previously discussed, it can be poor-functioning adrenals that are the real problem. An underactive thyroid gland (hypothyroidism) is not able to manufacture sufficient amounts of thyroid hormone. Thyroid hormone controls the metabolic rate of the body, the rate at which the cells convert food energy into physical energy (instead of depositing it as fat where you want your bikini line to be). An overactive thyroid is also a problem. Instead of being cold all the time and feeling sluggish, you are in hyperdrive and too warm, with an undue weight loss and potentially bulging eyes.

Both hypothyroidism and hyperthyroidism are problems. While there's no discounting hyperthyroidism, this section is going to focus on hypothyroidism. If you've picked up this book, it's more likely that of the two, it's a bigger concern for you.

What's the 411? The main thyroid hormones—TSH, T3, and T4—need to be in the right balance. One of the best steps you can undertake to keep your hormones in balance or heal them if they're "sick" is to decrease your overall stress level. Environmental factors, ingested toxins, and your emotional stressors can interfere with proper thyroid function. Go to Chapter 6. Read it forward and backward. Then read it again.

Most of us never received a lesson from our parents about how to think about stress properly. As a result, we don't have an adequate stress toolbox. We don't know how to work with stress well. There is no avoiding it. You're going to have stress. Seeing the effects that stress has on nearly every single hormone that either helps you have or robs you of energy should motivate you to revisit your stress toolbox.

Low thyroid function and low-level depression have similar effects on a woman as adrenal exhaustion. Check both your thyroid and your adrenal function and look at your lifestyle and nutrition before making a conclusion, together with a doctor, about starting any medications.

Always address the problem, not the symptom. Eating too little or too little of the right things, getting too little or too much exercise, and poor sleep habits are habits to correct first.

"Suboptimal" adrenal function doesn't test well. So, even if the fact that your adrenal glands are working overtime is the cause of your underactive thyroid, it will be hard to determine. Pay attention to your symptoms more than to the results of any testing you might undergo. How you feel never lies. Test, don't guess, is a good rule. On the other hand, tests don't always reveal the whole picture.

Dr. Christine Northrup, a leading authority on women's health, writes in her blog and Dr. Alan Christianson, in his book *The Adrenal Reset Diet*, concurs that though testing is possible, it is not always conclusive. If a low-functioning thyroid is present or suspected, then look first at your lifestyle habits and stress. Your symptoms don't lie. For example, say a test comes back, and you have normal levels of adrenal function. You still feel exhausted, right? Start reducing sugar in your diet. Increase your intake of organic foods and add natural herbs to your diet.

Dr. Northrup suggests adding a natural herbal remedy to your diet, such as Pueraria mirifica, maca, black cohosh, ground golden flaxseed, or chasteberry. Learn more about these possible remedies from your local health food store.

Dr. Christianson offers the following clarifying information on thyroid testing on his blog:

The most common approach is to run only a TSH blood test, and look at the TSH normal range. Many individuals would argue if you are above the range, then you have to check the T4 and see if it is below the range. By the most stringent, conventional guidelines, unless you have a severely elevated TSH (7 or greater) and a clearly low T4, there is no problem with your thyroid. So, that is the first thing not to do. The tests are actually really good, but the ranges are awful. Many people can have normal levels, but still have early thyroid disease.

- *You want to do a TSH test. You want to check the hormones released by the thyroid, as well. The TSH checks the pituitary, which tells the thyroid how to work. The hormones released include the T3 and T4. The free versions of those hormones are more meaningful than the total version. If it does not say anything besides just T3 or T4, this is the total version and not the free.*
- *It is also good to check for thyroid antibodies. If your body is attacking your thyroid, the gland typically gets diseased. So, you want to see if your body is attacking it. There is the thyroglobulin antibody (TG) and the thyroid peroxidase antibody (TPO).*
- *There is also thyroglobulin, which is not the antibody, just thyroglobulin. The presence of Thyroglobulin is a good measurement on how irritated or inflamed your thyroid is.*
- *You also want to check for reverse T3. Reverse T3 is a by-product of your body getting rid of T4, and this can be abnormal, as well.*
- *The last thing I encourage for those individuals who suspect thyroid disease is to get an ultrasound. There are many times when patients' labs are normal, or they don't have measurable antibodies, yet an ultrasound shows they have nodules, goiters, or calcifications, all clear signs of Hashimoto's.*

In terms of the labs, the one test that has the biggest difference in ranges from healthy populations to populations typically tested is the TSH test. Some individuals argue that the free hormones (like the free T3) should be on the higher end of the range. I do not see data to support that conclusion. The healthy populations show a large range of T3, as well as a large range of T4. They are not all in the upper end of the range. The TSH scores in the healthiest populations are at the lower end of the range. So, being on the lower end of the range means you're further away from being hypothyroid. Specifically, numbers above 1.9 are pretty suspicious. If your TSH is above 1.9, and you have some strong symptoms and some structural abnormalities, that's thyroid disease. It's time to treat it, so you can feel better.

Refer to the end of this chapter for additional advice from Dr. Christianson.

LEPTIN

Leptin, discovered in 1994, plays the role of "the starvation hormone," opposite ghrelin, which is starring as "the hunger hormone." You have an optimal leptin level, which is unique to you. When your leptin is below that level, your body senses starvation. It can happen when you diet, eat less, and lose weight. Your body, specifically your vagus nerve between your brain and abdomen, does everything it can to drive your level of leptin back up.

Either a low level of leptin or the presence of leptin resistance makes you hungrier. In other words, leptin functioning as it should at an optimal level would tell you when you're full and satisfied after a normal meal. Malfunctioning, it doesn't signal you to stop eating. It encourages you take in extra energy and store it as fat.

In overweight people, there is a large amount of leptin but the brain isn't getting the signal, aka "leptin resistance." Their leptin levels keep going higher. They're fat, but their brain can't see it. Their brain is starved, and their body is obese.

Since you want leptin to tell you when enough is enough, the question is what improves leptin function? Supplements aren't the answer. The leptin is there, but there's resistance to it. There are only about 100 documented cases in the world in which supplements have helped.

Leptin dysfunction is characterized by a number of factors, including the following:
- An increased desire to eat causes you to gain more weight.
- More body fat means more leptin in your fat cells.
- Too much fat means that proper leptin signaling is disrupted.
- Your brain thinks you're starving, which makes you want to eat more.
- You get fatter and hungrier.
- You eat more; you gain more weight.
- And so it continues … broken.

You can boost your level of leptin functioning in several ways, including the following:
- Decrease your level of insulin resistance by decreasing your intake of sugar.
- Decrease your level of triglycerides with moderate exercise and reduce your intake of simple sugars and processed foods.
- Reduce your intake of saturated fats, eliminate trans-fats, and increase your intake of healthy fats (omega 3s, fish oils).
- Limit your intake of alcohol.
- Maintain good gut health with prebiotics and probiotics, while reducing your intake of non-steroidal anti-inflammatory drugs (NSAIDS).

High lectin consumption, along with a lack of sleep, is tied to leptin dysfunction. While lectins are basically found in all foods, they exist in higher concentration in certain foods, including grains, especially wheat, soy legumes, nuts, dairy, eggplant, tomatoes, peppers, and genetically modified organisms (GMOs), to a lesser extent.

If leptin could be your problem, based on your lack of "full," then consider the following steps:

- Purge the worst offenders—grains and soy.
- Cut back on other offenders, such as dairy.
- Avoid GMOs.
- Maintain good gut health, e.g., reduce NSAIDS, eat probiotics and prebiotics, and consume good fats (fish oils).
- Consider not exercising, while you allow your body to heal and your hormones to rebalance over a period of a few weeks. An active lifestyle is good; just back off of your "workouts."
- If you do exercise, try it at night versus morning (this is opposite of cortisol) and focus on short bursts of exercise intervals and weight training, instead of long slow (dull) cardio, just for cardio's sake.
- Eat your meals at least four hours apart, and include protein in each meal, but avoid snacks. Let your body get things figured out. If you're truly hungry, that is a good sign. Four hours isn't too long between meals. Increase your intake of water. Also allow at least three to four hours between your last meal and bedtime.

Both ghrelin and leptin get messed up with obesity. There seems to be a high degree of variability. With weight gain, you'd expect your leptin levels to be low. They are often high, if you're dealing with leptin resistance. With weight gain, you'd expect your level of ghrelin to be low, while it may be high. Such a situation is often associated with a poor level of sleep.

On the other hand, in some obese subjects, the reverse is true. Sometimes, an individual experiences a complete lack of appetite, as well as a constant state of fullness, with or without physical activity. Activity doesn't always stimulate appetite. If you have put your body in starvation mode by eating too few calories for too long, it may need to recover. This factor is just one reason why, if you're obese, you may have "early satiety," in which you experience uncomfortable fullness on relatively little food. Possible solutions to this situation include reducing your intake of fiber and fat for a short period of time and eating smaller, frequent meals to let your body figure it out. Rule out other possible medical reasons for undue fullness by first checking with your physician.

GHRELIN

Ghrelin, which is known as *"the hunger hormone,"* was first discovered 1996, after leptin. Together, the two can have either a positive or negative effect on your appetite and therefore, on your ability to control your weight.

When your ghrelin levels are high, you're hungry or "hangry." If you get too little sleep, you could easily gain two pounds in as little as five days. Ghrelin increases your level of hunger and cravings, and then, leptin fails to tell you that you're full. Your body is cued up perfectly to store energy.

For the most part, this hormone-speak is biased toward how to overcome overweight, but underweight, or at least under-muscled, is also a problem as we age. For example, say you're relatively small. You have been on the thin side most of your life. As you age, you may find you're a "skinny fat." If you're losing muscle and don't have an appetite, ghrelin could have a positive effect on you.

The name ghrelin, in fact, is based on the hormone's role as a growth hormone-releasing substance. In other words, it can be good if you're losing muscle mass. It's not always the bad guy.

Ghrelin is a potent stimulator of growth hormone (GH) secretion and is the only circulatory hormone known to potently enhance appetite and weight gain and to regulate energy balance. Catabolic situations occur when you're losing muscle mass, and it's breaking down at a faster rate than its being repaired. Simple math says less muscle means more fat. A breakdown occurs more rapidly as we age. A breakdown happens after exercise. A breakdown takes place without enough protein and calories to repair and rebuild. If you're counting, that's three strikes you're out.

Furthermore, a rapid breakdown could come about due to illness or bed rest, for instance. In some women, a lack of appetite and the muscle losses that follow seem to ensue after relatively long periods of ignoring hunger signals. Ghrelin may enhance the appetite for better food intake, for increased gastric emptying, and heightened nutrient storage, coupled with an increase in GH. Muscle growth and repair processes would improve, which would help halt muscle losses. Some people are plagued, believe it or not, with a lack of appetite that physical activity doesn't help stimulate. Talk to your physician if this is you, no matter what your weight.

Ghrelin regulates your metabolism, primarily by affecting your food intake. If ghrelin is a problem, you will have more cravings and a bigger appetite, even when you physiologically don't need more fuel. As such, you will eat more, quite often of the wrong thing. Naturally, you're going to gain weight.

If you're constantly experiencing cravings, and you can tie it to missing your sleep quota, *then* start there. It's one of the most likely reasons that your level of ghrelin is higher. Even one poor night's sleep can increase your cravings—and typically you won't be craving kale and salmon.

ESTROGEN, PROGESTERONE, AND TESTOSTERONE

No discussion of hormones is complete without a mention of sex hormones. Estrogen levels typically go down post-menopause. Signs that you have a low estrogen level include hot flashes, night sweats, and dryer skin, eyes, and the big V.

Research from the University of Minnesota notes that foods that naturally help boost estrogen include apples, alfalfa, barley, baker's yeast, beets, cherries, chickpeas, carrots, celery, cucumbers, dates, fennel, oats, olives and olive oil, papaya, peas, plums, pomegranates, potatoes, beans, rhubarb, rice, tomatoes, wheat, and yams. Sesame seeds, flaxseed, and sunflower seeds have also been found to help to boost the levels of estrogen hormone in the body.

Herbs, especially chasteberry, can provide nutrition to glands that produce estrogen. Consult your physician for interactions with any other medications before taking.

Moderate exercise can help boost low estrogen levels, but overexercise can decrease estrogen levels. With regard to estrogen levels, don't compare yourself to your best friend forever (BFF) or anyone else. Focus on you, your symptoms, and your needs. The enjoyment of exercise is not always an indication that you should do more. Particularly if you feel flat when you exercise, you should consider taking a good break from it. If after a week of reduced exercise you're still experiencing high levels of stress, hot flashes, or weight gain, you need a short-term change to get you back to full function and your happy place. In this instance, a month of a much-reduced exercise schedule could be better for your efforts to lose weight and gain energy.

Your balance of estrogen and progesterone is important. Estrogen levels typically go down with menopause, making *estrogen dominance*, a potential obstacle in achieving weight loss a less common problem in older women. It's one to consider, however.

It all depends on cortisol. Do you see a theme here? Too much cortisol blocks progesterone, which means that your estrogen levels might be high *relative* to your level of progesterone. This imbalance causes problems. Your body can't fire on all cylinders, if everything isn't in good balance. If you're scoring well in all categories, but not getting results, look first to tame your cortisol-causing stress.

Eliminate high estrogen foods, like meat, temporarily if having a high estrogen level could be your issue. Focus on plants, beans, fish, and shellfish for protein. Eliminate sugars, a step that will also help you control your level of cortisol response.

Why is this a big deal at this point? You'd think fewer hormones, fewer problems. Estrogen and progesterone both have an anti-cortisol effect. Estrogen also has an anti-insulin effect. In other words, during pre-menopause, you have an easier time maintaining an hourglass shape. Your estrogen acts as a little insurance policy against the cortisol and insulin storm. Figuratively, when you lose the estrogen, your insurance policy is cancelled.

In order to stay sexy and vibrant, women need the right level of testosterone. Too low and you may feel lethargic, lack an appropriate level of sexual desire, or not enjoy yourself in the bedroom or otherwise. Having headaches or migraines can also be a symptom of low testosterone. *"I've got a headache"* is real. This factor ties to DHEA (refer to the next section for additional information), the precursor to testosterone. If your level of DHEA is low, the domino effect is low testosterone and the resulting low sex drive. On the other hand, if your level of testosterone is too high, belly fat is more likely. The need for balance prevails again.

The good news is that sex cures headaches.

DHEA

Dehydroepiandrosterone (DHEA or DHEA-S) is a naturally occurring weak androgenic steroid hormone, produced in both men and women by the adrenal glands that helps prevent aging, improves sexual function, enhances athletic performance, and facilitates the treatment of osteoporosis. DHEA is a very powerful precursor to all of the major sex hormones—estrogen, progesterone, and testosterone. All factors considered, it needs to be present and accounted for in order for the optimal level of the three sex hormones to exist. We've discussed the other three hormones in the previous section. If needed, DHEA can convert to testosterone, provided, of course, that your DHEA is not compromised.

DHEA is another hormone swinger. It can be too high or too low and cause problems. Too much DHEA has been associated with acne and depression in menopause. Higher DHEA increases insulin resistance in many menopausal women. Keep in mind that when insulin sensitivity is a problem for you, both insulin and cortisol are going to make you store fat much easier.

A 2014 study found that an elevated level of DHEA is mitigated by exercise. In other words, although exercise won't make your DHEA go down, your level of insulin sensitivity will improve. Things are better balanced. How much exercise did it take? Study subjects did six days of 60 minutes of combined weight and aerobic training a week for six months. (Daily weight training required that different muscle groups were rotated between workouts.)

Remember that besides DHEA, your adrenals also produce the stress hormones cortisol and adrenaline. *Adrenal exhaustion* occurs from coping with chronic stress—from, among other things, poor nutrition, yo-yo dieting, emotional turmoil, and job-related stress. In other words, your adrenals are pooped from pumping out cortisol and they simply can't manufacture enough DHEA to support a healthy hormonal balance. If your level of cortisol is high and your DHEA is low, then, you feel tapped out, overwhelmed, and, often, depressed. Bad combination.

Achieving a balance between your levels of cortisol and DHEA should be a goal for you. (Doesn't it seem that cortisol needs some lessons in getting along well with others?) When your adrenal glands aren't functioning properly, it means that your cortisol is too high relative to your DHEA. Again, with the balance. At any moment, you're about to think you're having a senior moment, and you've already read this part before. If this is starting to feel like a Rubik's Cube, when you get one side perfectly aligned and another is then screwed up, you've got it!

In all likelihood, at some point in your life, you've seen someone solve a Rubik's Cube. This hormone balance puzzle is solvable too. The point to remember is that nothing about you works independently. Take off the blinders about masochist calorie burning at the altar of the boot camp and starving in order to lose weight. Imagine those steps as leading you to drive faster and faster in the wrong direction.

When your DHEA levels are good you have improved energy, vitality, sleep, and better mental clarity. If pre-menstrual syndrome has been a problem, you'll have reduced PMS, and recover more optimally from acute stress or trauma. DHEA, along with growth hormone, can help you keep that muscle mass. It balances the negative effects of cortisol.

DHEA levels drop in part of the aging process in some women. You make about 25 mg of DHEA per day (more or less), with typically dwindling production, as you get older. Men at all ages have more DHEA than women. If you need it, DHEA supplementation for adrenal support could make a big difference.

One study found three months of daily supplementation of 50 mg DHEA increased DHEA levels in study participants to that of young adults. Subjects reported a marked increase in their physical and psychological well-being. Dr. Daniel Amen in his book, *Unleash the Power of the Female Brain,* suggests a metabolite of DHEA called 7-Keto-DHEA that can have fewer side effects (acne and facial hair) than DHEA.

You may be tempted to reach for the DHEA available over-the-counter. Popping DHEA alone won't do you any good if your adrenals are exhausted. It's all about integration. Don't guess about supplements. Test and retest, along with consulting with your physician.

Supplementation, if needed, is temporary. Once you're back in balance, there's no need to continue with DHEA supplementation. Accordingly, the solution is easy—and fun. Find joy! People with a positive outlook actually create a self-sustaining cycle of DHEA production. As such, they produce more DHEA, which may also affect their levels of serotonin (happiness neurotransmitter). In turn, they have a better outlook, which ups their level of DHEA, and so on. This is the end of the vicious cycle and the beginning of the happy dance.

How do you test the status of your adrenal function, DHEA, and cortisol? Saliva adrenal profiles can be used. Total cortisol levels aren't going to show up well on these tests, however. How you feel doesn't lie. Listen to your body. If you've learned too well to ignore your symptoms, start tuning in again. At that point, ask yourself if the changes you've made in your nutrition, exercise, and sleep have made a difference? Is there still a disconnect between how you feel and the positive changes that you've made?

If you've made changes according to this book, having unlearned some old habits and let go of old thoughts, but still aren't finding results, it's time to talk to your physician.

If you suspect adrenal imbalance, hormonal imbalance, or a DHEA irregularity, your physician can order an adrenal panel. Using blood tests, she'll check your estrogen, progesterone, and your DHEA, as well as both your free and total testosterone levels at appropriate stages in your cycle. You want estrogen, progesterone, and DHEA in the upper quadrant of normal. When a "range of health" is given for test results, realize being *just inside the limit* could indicate a problem.

Your symptoms don't lie. Tune in and trust your symptoms. Normal should be happiness, stable energy, feeling rested after a good night's sleep, and a healthy sex drive. That's not too much to ask. If you have a few pounds to lose, and are at the starting line of your efforts in this regard and these qualities describe your life, you're not far from your optimal weight for health.

If, on the other hand, that's not your picture of health right now, don't jump into a diet or extreme exercise. Set yourself up for success with happier hormones first.

FEATURED EXPERT

Dr. Alan Christianson

❏ One Trick to Improve Your Adrenal and Thyroid Hormones

Think of the thyroid gland as a dynamo that generates massive amounts of electricity by water flowing through a dam. In this analogy, the adrenal glands would be the switch that allows this electricity to leave the dam and travel down the wires, where it will be used by neighboring homes.

Thyroid hormones give energy to your body, allowing it to burn fuel and do work. This energy is also needed for the repair of your tissues, like your skin, hair, and nails. When this energy is lacking, you feel tired. You also might feel less mentally sharp, and/or more depressed, or rundown. Because you're not able to burn the fuel you feed your body, it all gets stored as fat. This situation is the double-whammy of gaining weight and being tired at the same time. You would think that storing energy would make you feel more energized, but the opposite is true. It is a physical sign that your body is not properly burning energy. Instead, it is storing too much of it.

Because these thyroid hormones are so powerful, your body has many ways to regulate them. The main way is by regulating how much hormone comes out of your thyroid gland and goes into your circulation. This factor is called the central control of thyroid hormones. The other main way these hormones are regulated is called peripheral control, which includes all of the things that happen in your body after the hormones have already been released. Of all of the peripheral control steps, none is more powerful than the adrenal hormones, especially cortisol.

Every single part of your body is made up of individual cells. These cells include your hair, brain, skin, bones, muscles, nerves, organs, and nails. All of these cells need just the right amount of thyroid hormones to work properly.

These cells are all surrounded by cell membranes, which is kind of like the walls and doors in your house. Just like a door, these membranes control what is allowed to enter the cell and what is kept out.

In order for the doors to open and let thyroid hormones inside, cortisol has to hit the doorbell on a regular basis, but not too much. In states of health, cortisol is made in higher amounts in the morning, which allows your body to be alert and active when your cells are absorbing all the thyroid hormones. Later in the day, this process reverses, and cortisol shuts down. This shutdown of cortisol lets you get deep, refreshing sleep, and repair all of your aches and pains, which helps get your body ready for another busy productive day.

When these two glands are working together well, your body will produce abundant energy all throughout the day. You will also be able to effortlessly maintain a healthy, lean body weight, without having to micromanage every morsel of food you consume.

What is one easy thing you can do today to help your thyroid and adrenals give you great energy and great metabolism? Be strategic about your caffeine usage. Foods that contain caffeine happen to have pigments called anthocyanins that are very strong in healing antioxidants. This factor is why there have been many health news stories extolling the benefits of caffeinated beverages. It is important, however, to realize that the benefits come from the anthocyanins, not from the caffeine.

People have very significant differences on how well they can tolerate caffeine. It is also true that we all become more sensitive to caffeine once we pass our mid 20s. Specifically what happens is that it takes longer to move caffeine through our liver and out of our body as we age. If you are in your 40s, you might be able to eliminate up to 100 mg of caffeine over the course of the day. Imagine what would happen if you consumed even just 120 mg every day. Rather than starting over each day, you would have a backlog left over from the day before, on top of the extra hundred 120 mg that day. The problem is that eventually you have caffeine in your bloodstream all day long, even if you only consume it in the morning.

That continual exposure to caffeine prevents you from shutting off your cortisol at night. For many people, that can lead to poor quality sleep, harder to get to sleep, and harder to stay asleep. You can also prevent your body from responding to your thyroid hormones in the morning, which makes you more tired and less able to burn fat.

If you are a regular caffeine user, among the ways to be strategic about it are the following:
- Take a minimum of one day per week to avoid caffeine altogether. This schedule will keep you from building up a backlog. For many individuals,

two days can work even better, especially when they are consecutive. Here's a secret: the days you have caffeine, you will enjoy it more and get more of a boost out of it than you would if you were a daily user.

- If you are more sensitive to caffeine than others, you may be better off focusing on decaffeinated beverages, like coffee or tea. Some individuals are sensitive enough to where they are better off avoiding even decaffeinated beverages on a regular basis. Keep in mind that "decaffeinated" does not mean caffeine-free.

Want to learn more about your adrenal glands? Check out our free quizzes on www.adrenalquiz.com to learn what your adrenal glands are doing and how you can help them further!

Alan Christianson is a New York Times' bestselling author and a Phoenix, Arizona-based naturopathic medical doctor (NMD), who specializes in natural endocrinology, with a focus on thyroid disorders. He is the author of The Adrenal Reset Diet, The Complete Idiot's Guide to Thyroid Disease, *and* Healing Hashimoto's: A Savvy Patient's Guide.

He frequently appears on national TV, including Dr. Oz, CNN, The Doctors, *and the* Today *show, as well as in print media like* Women's World, USA Today, Newsweek, *and* Shape *magazine. When he's not maintaining a busy practice, his favorite hobbies include mountain unicycling, technical rock climbing, and watching the stars. Dr. Christianson resides in Scottsdale, Arizona with his wife, Kirin, and their two children.*

The doctor of the future will give no medicines, but will interest his patients in the care of the human frame, in diet, and in the causes and prevention of disease.

—Thomas Edison

CHAPTER 9 ———————

A Whole-You Plan

You're there. This is the future. There is no more talking about your mind, body, and soul in isolation. You're the complete package.

This is the whole enchilada. Be reminded that this text isn't a fitness book based on simple exercise prescription and optimal nutrition. A "diet" and a "workout" aren't going to do it. If you are a "normal" after 50 fox, you have a library of those books already by now, and another one won't make a difference.

The goal is to look at what's going haywire with your smoking-hot, second-50 plan and adjust to a strategy that actually works, instead of one that ignores your changing needs. The trends, fads, and the logical exercise prescription for a body with balanced hormones will send you further off balance, if you're teetering on the menopause or stress high wire. The old patterns of behavior and thoughts you learned aren't going to work in this new game. The rules have changed.

Be clear, however. You don't need a soft approach, because you're getting old. You need a different approach, because your hormones and your mindset are messing with you. You need to align them, and then, you can work as hard as you want, as well as achieve the level of fitness and energy that you want. You can walk into the closet and wear what you want. You can walk into a room and get heads turning, if you want.

You may have always been active. At this point, however, you're aware that you're not in your 20s, and you need a different set of rules. You may not have ever exercised or watched what you ate. You describe your diet as "healthy." Maybe, you were naturally thin, or you simply didn't make the time before this point. You now know that you want something different for the years ahead. No matter what's prompted you to read this book, you have an opportunity to make the rest of your years the best of your years.

If you're looking for an excuse to slow down and settle for inactivity and weight gain, while you age, this book will have been light reading and entertainment at best. Decide right now not to be your own biggest obstacle. Wanting change and committing to making the daily changes necessary to get it are two different things.

You may not be able to exercise the way you'd like to right now. You still have six other lifestyle areas that significantly impact your results. The truth of your reality is in the blurb on the front cover of this book: *Eat More, Exercise Less, Heal Hormones, and Boost Energy for Whole-You Wellness.* Less exercise gets better results than more for more's sake. If you don't love exercise, you can still be in amazing shape. If you do love exercise, you'll have an easier time making adjustments to what you're doing so well already.

There has never been a better time to be in your second 50. Enjoy it. Get to the end of your life's journey saying, *what a ride!*

Once you've read this final chapter, decide which chapter topic is most associated with the hormone change you need. Start there. Do you need to reread the chapter on hormones, or have you narrowed it down to nutrition, exercise, stress, or sleep being the best place for you to start? Signs and symptoms you're experiencing connect you to the hormone-balancing action or inaction that will be the most beneficial for you. Use the appendices and your checklist scores to guide you. Start planning your nutrition, exercise, sleep, rest, and stress-enhancing strategies one-by-one. Begin with your one most important change for positive hormone balance. You'll naturally integrate the others into your plan.

The whole-you approach means that you don't just blindly do a workout, because it's on the calendar today. You respond to your stressors, sleep, and energy levels. The curves that life throws at you require that whatever plan you create needs flexibility. There will be days when the best thing for you is to exchange doing high-intensity intervals for a yoga class or a walk in nature.

There will be overlap. If you identify sleep deprivation as contributing to your cortisol problems, your nutrition plan may be equally important in helping you get more sleep. By now, you are aware that the hormone chaos caused by sleep loss will make you more vulnerable to cravings. You'll need to follow the steps previously discussed to plan for that. You want improvement in sleep that occurs from changing not only your sleep habits, but also your nutrition. Exercise type and timing can help sleep hygiene as well. Those specific changes may be different than your BFF's unique plan.

Review the following highlights from each of the early chapters. The *After 50 Fitness Formula* case studies and success stories used in this chapter and earlier in the book are all based on real clients. While the names, in most cases, have been changed, the details are real. The case studies are included to help you see how to create a personal plan. This author would love to hear from you as you do it. Please use the contact information in the back of the book or visit http://foreverfitandfab.com.

NUTRITION

Your food is either medicine or poison. The type, the timing, and the amount you need vary, based on your hormone needs. Your optimal hormone-balancing nutrition plan may deviate from traditional RDAs. Your gut health and food sensitivities require a nutrition plan that is like a thumbprint—uniquely yours.

Either a lack of calories or a lack of the right type of calories is often the biggest downfalls of women over 50. You may have years of thoughts and patterns to unlearn. Dieting places stress on the body, which brings you back to cortisol-caused problems. If, on the other hand, you include sweet fruits, wine, and desserts regularly in your diet, insulin could be your challenge. Identify your biggest symptoms—something's not right. Connect that to your habits. Then strategize.

Regularly limiting your calories sends your body the message to burn fewer calories. This approach is a fat-belly formula. You've done it. You're at lunch pouring over a menu, and if the calorie count is there, you zoom in on it and change your mind, instead of ordering what you really want. If you're choosing between a salmon entrée and a green salad without protein, that math doesn't work.

At this point in your life, an excess of belly fat is not a permanent state of affairs. You can improve your metabolism at any age. Turn your back on calories, and head toward nutrient-dense foods that balance hormones. Build meals and snacks around lean protein sources and healthy (omega 3) fats. Fill in first with vegetables, then lower GL fruits, and last, grains that work for your body.

Sugar, from all its obvious and hidden sources, influences insulin. Together with cortisol, that is also a belly-fat formula. You can have your cake. Don't think that because you're accepting a lifestyle change, that you're going down a path void of cream-cheese frosting or chocolate. Wash your mouth out with soap! You just have to strategically plan those treats at times when the negative impact on your body is low.

While even temporary removal of some foods, coffee, or wine may seem incredibly hard, you can do it. Nicotine, for example, is a very addictive substance. Women who smoke can give it up when they're pregnant, even though many start again after delivery. You've done a fasting blood test and forgone the coffee, bedtime snack, and breakfast. Maybe, you've had the backdoor checked and done bland food for days in preparation. You can do this too. The harder you think it is, the more likely you're going to benefit. Do you just like that afternoon soda or are you addicted to it?

If you truly have disordered thoughts about food, and you know it, seek help. Dysfunctional thinking about food is common and complex. You probably don't recognize your own irrational thoughts about food. Trust someone you know for insight. If you operate with a lot of strict "rules" related to food, talk to someone about how it could be negatively affecting your health. If you think you "eat healthy," and the eyes staring back at you aren't twinkling, the skin isn't glowing, or you don't have the energy to burn, you deserve all those things. Check it out.

You can exchange fat-phobia and calorie counting for a lean body. It's possible, if you can change the six inches between your ears. Start small. Approach change step-by-step and build confidence. For example, increase the amount of lean protein you have each meal first. Next, focus on including a healthy fat at each meal and snack. Then, increase the amount of fiber you ingest daily. The best way to approach nutrition change is to focus on all that you can have, rather than what you can't.

This very next sentence will appear to contradict the previous one. Go through the elimination diet. If you're a lifetime dieter, you just got excited. You're good at this. You can do this, you're thinking. Stop. This is not your mother's diet. You're not reducing calories or enduring hunger pains with the elimination diet. It's about exchanging foods that you may be sensitive to for ones that you're not. Pay attention to your desire to go on a "diet." If it still lingers, thoughts that there is a quick fix still exist for you. That will get in the way of you living your life to the fullest, at your leanest and most energetic self. For suggestions on how to go through the elimination diet—eliminating as many toxins as possible—refer to the elimination diet journal and *14-Day Double Your Energy Undiet* link in Appendix A-3.

AFTER 50 INSPIRATION: TERI WARD

❏ *"I want to get faster and stronger."*

During Teri Ward's 45-minute interview, not once did weight, diet, or appearance come up. In the brief time dedicated to talk about training, there was more discussion about the benefits of meditation, Pilates, and yoga than burning calories.

Sixty-two-year-old Teri Ward says she was in her 50s when she really first got active. Playing tennis and golf regularly, she had a scare when she couldn't keep up with a group, while hiking. She subsequently booked an appointment with her doctor. The diagnosis?

❏ *"You're out of shape."*

So, at age 57, living in the triathlon mecca of the world, without a bike or swim skills, Teri decided it was time to tri. The multisport appeal of swimming, biking, and running struck Teri as a balanced approach to fitness.

Her first bike came from craigslist. Her first swim, as luck would have it, introduced her to what would be an age-group friend on a similar path.

Teri tri-ed her way from short to long distances, cumulating at competing at Ironman in Boulder, Colorado in 2015. Her five-year venture into triathlon wasn't without a hiccup, however. An injury from skiing sidelined her for three months, until finally she resorted to a steroid injection. One shot and she was pain-free, and on her way to a season of races that led to her registering for the 140.2 mile Ironman just 18 months later.

"I was told that I couldn't do stuff. Nobody can tell me I can't now," Teri says of growing up in an era before this new generation of movers.

The Grace to Race, a book about iron nun Madonna Buder, inspired Teri. Buder started her running career at 46, and, by age 80, had completed 340 triathlons, 45 of them Ironman distance. Both Teri at 62 and Buder at 85 are still going strong.

Teri's questions to herself now are about lifting limits, not imposing them. *"What are my limits? Do I have any? Or is it in my head?"* she asks. Indeed.

Note: If you're wondering how this inspirational brief fits into the "exercise less" concept, the author had the same pause. Yet, Teri didn't start with miles and hours. She started small. Careful and progressive training works. At 55, she never dreamed of doing an Ironman. At this point in her life, she wouldn't dream of a different lifestyle. What haven't you dreamed yet?

EXERCISE

Find your sweet spot. If cortisol-causing exercise is all you're doing regularly, you need to take a break. Look at the total stress load in your life. Look at signs that what you're doing is not working. If you simply go on with your demanding workouts expecting that more of what got you here in the first place will make things better, you're running fast in the wrong direction.

When things in your life were less stressful and going well, you may have gotten away with frequently placing high-intensity exercise (either short intervals or long duration endurance) demands on your body. You may again. Right now, though, if you're not sleeping, you're not losing weight, you're exhausted, instead of energized, and you don't have a formula that's working. The more stressors piled on your plate, the less able your body is to recover. Something's gotta give. For you, it may mean you need to move more or less. You may need to exchange high intensity for low intensity or vice versa. This personal exercise plan doesn't fit well into a boot-camp biology. Create your own needs list before you go shopping for a program. Do that by identifying what's not working, instead of what results you want.

Look at each day in both isolation and integration with the others. Busy day? Lighten the exercise load. A day off or simply a lighter day will fit better at this point for you. Busy month? Put off that half-marathon goal right now. If taking time for your walk or yoga is foreign to you, find a friend or pay a trainer to hold you accountable.

If insulin has deposited belly fat around your middle, exercise can act as an excellent blood-sugar stabilizer. You don't have to start with boot camp six days a week. A short walk, most days of a week, is a start. Movement most days punctuated by higher intensity on some days is a reasonable goal. Both too little or too much exercise can let your hormone divas run the show.

Embrace the idea that exercise is not your first line of defense against hormones. You heard it from a fitness professional first. Removing it from the equation may reduce the noise in your life and allow you to hear what else is going on. You may need blinders to avoid the messages telling you to move more and push harder. At this point in your life, if you're exercising and eating "right," but not seeing or feeling results, your body is telling you that your hormone exercise prescription needs to be very different than the textbook one an exercise instructor might be throwing at you.

INSPIRING AFTER 50: DEBBI, AKA MIDDLE AGED TRIATHLETE

Depending on how you use it, Facebook can be a source of motivation or discouragement. Examples of people living life right now in its perfect imperfection can help you get over, around, and through your litany of excuses. One source of motivation can be found at www.facebook.com/MiddleAgedTryathlete.

Even at first glance, Debbi Segina's first triathlon at 58 is very impressive. She had a total hip replacement at 57. Most people don't consider triathlon training traditional as rehab for total hip replacement.

Debbi's story doesn't end there. Actually, it didn't start there. There's more. More is a cancer diagnosis at age 24. This 36-year cancer survivor has always been a fighter. Faced with choosing a wheelchair or hip surgery, she didn't blink.

Triathlon is not the first choice of most total-hip replacement patients or their surgeons. Swimming and biking posed no problem, but running is not recommended. The shelf life of a bionic hip has limits. The warranty expires, if you're going to run on it.

Debbi's exercise was prompted by her need to lose weight to take pressure off her joints and increase her level of mobility. What began as a tentative first visit to a small running group that welcomed walkers—even those with an 18-minute mile—has become a lifestyle.

Debbi's first sprint triathlon occurred after competing in 5Ks and short running races. The next goal on her training plan is an Olympic-distance tri, and she's entertaining the possibility of an Ironman. She doesn't train full time. In fact, maybe like you, she has a commute on each end of her workday of over an hour. It's not convenient for her to exercise.

Following doctor's orders, Debbi doesn't run, she walks. Get out of the way when you see her coming though. Her personal record for walking is just over a 12-minute mile.

Don't underestimate the power of the human spirit. When you look for excuses, you'll find them. When you look for answers, you'll also find them.

Listen to the WellU After 50 podcast with Debbi from May 12, 2015: https://itunes.apple.com/us/podcast/welluafter50-podcast/id903871206?mt=2

STRESS

If you have toxic stress, your hormone albatross is definitely cortisol. You may be crossing the menopausal divide. If so, estrogen got your attention. Cortisol is still the one hormone that is causing you all the trouble. Think about one change you could make that would make your life less stressful. It's potentially so obvious that you can't see it, like you can't see your nose on your face.

Women who suffer most from stress are caregivers and service providers, who've put themselves last for far too long. On the other hand, agreeing that you need to put your oxygen mask on first and doing it are two very different things.

If you don't have great stress skills, you're not alone. You're exposed to more stress environmentally, socially, and physically than any generation before you. If you're a caregiver by nature or nurture, you're more prone to feelings of guilt or for a need for permission to take care of yourself. Permission granted.

You may be tempted to reach for tangible actions. Resist the temptation to add a sudden change in your diet and exercise levels to your already elevated stress levels. Focus on one change that is manageable. Small and simple habits that reduce stress do matter. Create a new habit by coupling it with something that you already do. Take 10 deep breaths outdoors each time you eat a meal. Add a yoga class with a friend once a week, or instead get an exercise DVD and do the routine on it in your living room before you have dinner.

Remind yourself that though yoga or slow walking isn't a calorie-burning way to lose fat, you won't feel any less stressed or have more energy if you lose weight or fat in a quick fix way. If your hormones aren't balanced, your optimal weight, as well as your energy, will not come back. Gone to Tahiti. Do the foundational work you need to do first. If you reach for calorie-torching exercise or undertake calorie-slashing first, your body will suffer from more stress. You will still be stressed if you are ignoring the things that need to be said, the irrational thoughts that need to be addressed, or the too many hours spent in front of a screen. While you confront your stressors, add the healing power of nature, laughter, music, or your personal stress toolkit. There's no getting around this one. Ignoring your stress will not make it go away.

Consider including only light activity, preferably outdoors, first. Avoid strenuous workouts initially. Then, engage in short-in-duration sessions and keep those restricted to the morning. Next, add weight training. If you're stressed, you're probably not having sex, which by itself, adds more stress. Testosterone levels are positively affected by weight training. A little testosterone does a girl and her partner good. Activity in the weight room can boost your fun in the bedroom.

Identify the cravings triggered by stress and avoid bringing those foods into your house. Make it easy to do the right thing. Spinach, kale, and a bit of dark chocolate can help heal your stress. Packaged, processed, and high-carbohydrate foods have a negative impact on your stress levels. Traditional "comfort food" consumption induces a coma, not comfort.

SLEEP

Sleep deprivation either starts with your stress level or contributes to it. The exercise and nutritional strategies that apply to stress also apply to sleep. In essence, cortisol is the diva responsible for all of the problems again. Keep moderate-to-vigorous exercise to the morning. Make appropriate modifications in your exercise routine, if you've lost over two hours of sleep. For example, don't challenge yourself with activities that involve balance and coordination on these days. You're more likely to come up injured than fit.

Sleep is your first step. Only then will you have the potential to really feel good and make wise choices about nutrition. Remember that as little as a loss of two hours sleep begins to mimic being under the influence. How well do you make food choices when you're drunk?

Focus on your sleep hygiene. Look at your relationship with sleep. If you've had insomnia for years, you may avoid going to bed because you toss and turn. It's like your association with a dentist, if you've had lots of work done. Start looking at new high thread-count sheets or changing the color in your room to one that is soothing and relaxing. Find a book or a magazine you love and look forward to reading. Keep it for before bedtime only, so that you have something to look forward to when it's time to go to bed. Create positive associations with sleep.

REST AND RECOVERY

Rest and recovery is closely connected to both your exercise plan and your stress level. It can also be interlinked with your past dietary habits. Regardless of the factor, you often need recovery from too much. Too much exercise, too much dietary restriction, too much toxic exposure from either your food, environment, or a relationship gone bad all require recovery.

In Western societies, there's no reward for rest. When Westerners visit European cultures, where business halts mid-afternoon so everyone can take a siesta, they're often puzzled or frustrated.

You're rewarded for what you get done and what you produce. Too often, you're rewarded for the long hours of dedication you put in. Productivity and time commitment are two different things. The premise that thinking time and effort equals results reinforces overwork and suggests that anything less is something you should feel guilty about. At a minimum, if you don't have anything to show for your time, you at least logged long hours, right? It's easy to associate self-worth with doing more. Results, though, are always what matter most.

This factor is true both in the business world and in the business of your fitness. More strategically planned rest and recovery will lead to more optimal results. If you've starved yourself for months or years from real rest, you may need a big dose of it for a while. It will be hard. The little diva in your head may tell you that you're lazy. You might have withdrawals, particularly if you're really addicted to adrenalin. The very thing that causes your stress can be what "juices" you. It's your crack.

Breaking this cycle, even though it is clearly not working for you, will be like getting off a drug. Let the rehab begin.

HORMONES

For a review on hormones that may be stealing the starring role in your story, refer to Chapter 8. The big players are woven into the previous paragraphs. Based on what you've just read, you should have a good idea of where to begin. Some factors, like cortisol, have a cascade effect on others.

Resist your urge to start applying *all* of the tips and insights you've just learned. New Year's resolutions usually fail because they attempt to tackle everything at once.

AFTER 50 FITNESS STRATEGIES: KAREN

Karen showed up for coaching with a crazy sleep schedule and a propensity for going to bed shortly after her late night meal. In the mornings, she would wake but stay in bed, describing the period as the only time she relaxed. Then, she was off to the gym—maybe with a handful of almonds—often exercising so intensely for at least an hour that she had a recurring foot problem that had hung on for nearly a year.

She was following a mostly Paleo diet. After exercise, she would head to her home office and computer, working up to nine more hours, often without post-exercise fuel and skipping lunch. Then, she'd wind down her day late in the evening with a few cocktails, followed by a full dinner at 9 p.m. and bed by 11. Rinse and repeat.

Karen had previously lost a significant amount of weight. She regained part of it after a year and was concerned about regaining more. She couldn't figure out how she wasn't losing weight, given all she was doing.

What was happening to Karen? Cortisol was having a party and had invited insulin over as soon as the highball glasses came out. From there, the two stored the fat for another day. Taxed adrenal glands left Karen fatigued, stressed, wired, and unable to really get any restorative sleep.

Mentally, she was a wreck. She was under stress to earn more and build her business. Because a creative mind works when it wants to, pulling away from her design work to eat took a back seat to projects.

While she was disciplined about exercise and desperate to lose weight, she kept herself on that roller coaster of hard and long exercise, as well as starving her body before bingeing. Her meal in the evening wasn't truly a binge, but her body would treat it like it was, since it had to go for so long with so many mental, emotional, and physical stressors that it was primed to store fat instead of nourishing itself with the meal. A schedule of following hours of no food with alcohol shut down Karen's fat metabolism and sealed fat in the vault.

To break this cycle, Karen was asked to add a healthy meal after morning exercise and shift her dinner (without alcohol) and bedtime routine to two to three hours earlier. If she ate by 7 p.m. and was in bed by 10 p.m., she could rise easier. By six in the morning, she would have had eight hours of quality sleep (unlike the type of sleep that results following the consumption of alcohol) and be able to correct her circadian rhythm. Her sleep would have a restorative quality. Her exercise would have more positive impact on her, if she shortened it on most days and then went outdoors for light exercise and sunlight on recovery days. A chronic injury is a sign something is breaking down and your system is not working.

That's a lot of change at once. So, where did Karen start? What was the one thing that was going to have the greatest impact on Karen's success? Cortisol. You need to make that cortisol diva play the way you want her to play. A week entirely off from exercise, but including active breaks from work, and taking walks outdoors was a first step for Karen. Reintroducing short-duration, high-intensity exercise three to four mornings a week was next for her. This step allowed Karen to get the activity she loved—and get out of her home-office—without digging a deeper hole. Two of those days are cardio, and two are resistance training. On the other days, Karen should get outdoors for light walks or bike rides, either in the morning or instead of consuming a cocktail in the afternoon. The morning sunshine would be very helpful in resetting Karen's sleep clock.

Exercise will feel like less work with a light snack that has both carbohydrate and protein. Instead of the hard-to-digest almonds, a small bit of almond butter on a banana or a small smoothie with whey would be easy to digest. After exercise, a protein-rich meal before she dives into work would boost her muscle recovery and prevent muscle loss that can occur at age 54. It also increases focus and productivity. Instead of hours on end in front of a computer, edgy with brain fog, a relaxed constant expenditure of energy gets more done in less time.

Karen was playing a big willpower game and losing. She was operating on adrenaline and discipline, while concurrently depriving herself of nutrients and calories during the day. By evening, she felt she needed a reward. The alcohol and eating whatever she wanted made sense to her by then. She wasn't doing this on purpose, but it was a habit she had to change in order to lose weight and get her energy back.

Karen had been ignoring her hunger and put herself into starvation mode on a daily basis. In that instance, the body is much more likely to store fat when it actually gets fuel. Cortisol and insulin were sabotaging any positive steps that Karen was taking. It takes time for the body to heal itself from that kind of habitual eating, but it can happen successfully at any age.

AFTER 50 FITNESS STRATEGIES: ROBYN

Robyn answered her new client intake, saying, "We eat really healthy." That's usually a red flag. It means, *I eat the way I personally define as healthy, even though I may not be getting the results I want.* Beliefs about what is healthy come from a history of growing up in the diet-rich environment in which you existed.

Many boomer women voice good intentions about eating healthy. In Robyn's case, she was exhausted, stressed, not sleeping well, and had gained weight around the middle, in spite of a long history of engaging in physical activity.

For the most part, *healthy* for Robyn meant no meat. No snacking. Regular vigorous exercise before long stressful days running her own business was her habit. She liked order and routine. It's how she got things done every day. Then, it was back home to walk her dogs briskly, drink wine, and eat dinner void of protein or featuring texturized protein in frozen vegan or vegetarian patties.

Very infrequently, she had higher quality protein from eggs (with turkey sausage) for breakfast. For both the mental and physical energy she poured into her very full life, Robyn wasn't getting enough nutrients. Few vegetables, little fruit, few fats, and random protein were Robyn's nutritional norm. There were few antioxidant and inflammation-reducing foods in her diet. Yet, there were several inflammation-causing toxins, including her computer screen and her always plugged in lifestyle. Robyn's personal to-do list was long.

Robyn wanted weight loss, especially around her belly, as well as more energy. She'd always prided herself on her appearance and active lifestyle.

Lately, though, she wasn't getting anywhere. Robyn's first step was to increase the number of regular meals she consumed. Robyn was wearing braces that made eating during the day a challenge, since popping braces out for a snack seemed a huge inconvenience. She introduced a liquid shake to her diet, with protein, veggies, and small amounts of berries added. A made-from-home liquid shake, with real spinach or fruit, was optimal, but if all else failed, a pre-packaged, low-sugar or stevia-sweetened protein drink was better than nothing. Robyn was asked to increase her consumption of fish and ground turkey for the high-quality protein she needed, but wasn't getting from texturized processed proteins.

Stabilizing her level of blood sugar, with regularly spaced meals, and increasing her level of satiety with healthy fats were a start. Increasing more slow-digesting carbs at her evening meal supported Robyn's brisk walk with her dogs and helped enhance the quality and the amount of her sleep. Wine, she had to learn, was not a food group. Wine should be reserved for special occasions, and then not on an empty stomach after a stressful day, during which it would increase her level of insulin and halt her level of fat metabolism.

Her sleep quality improved dramatically within a few weeks. As a business owner, with a great deal of discipline, it took a lot of convincing for Robyn to realize that she could make an executive decision and start later. That way, she could begin her day with the exercise that was important to her and start with a good breakfast, instead of having to choose one over the other.

Take time to examine the self-talk you're doing. It can play a part in reducing the effects of cortisol on you. Who doesn't have irrational thoughts? The problem is, when you're having them, you don't recognize it. That's what makes it irrational! Robyn had a long list of things that just had to get done, even on her days off work. Ask yourself, "What if that car doesn't get washed or the laundry doesn't all get done?" Come up with laughable answers, and you can lighten your load, as well as your level of cortisol.

AFTER 50 FITNESS STRATEGIES: DOROTHY

Dorothy is a giver. Her nursing job is all about serving others and putting them first. Her goals were weight loss, as well as, ultimately, to feel better about herself. She had started to turn down vacation opportunities with her friends. The thought of a swimsuit being the dress code and consuming cocktails and food that she knew wasn't on a "diet" were a turn-off.

She doesn't love to exercise. She didn't know what to do. She's never really had a consistent habit of exercising, but when she was most active, she enjoyed group-fitness classes. When she gets busy or has a bad night's sleep, which is frequently, exercise is the first to go.

A lack of nutrition knowledge and lingering beliefs about dieting were getting in the way of Dorothy's progress. She often resorted to packaged and processed foods, marketed as "healthy," that she'd find on the shelves at Costco. Her first attempts at choosing healthier foods involved high-carbohydrate, high-sugar foods. She didn't have any level of awareness about how different foods affected her body or metabolism. She was used to barely eating during long, stressful days at work and, then, rewarding herself with popcorn and snacks in front of the TV at night.

In the morning, she wasn't hungry so she'd skip breakfast. She might find something—usually not very nutritious—in the breakroom, if she got hungry. Then, she'd not have much more to eat until evening. She woke frequently at night and never felt rested. In reality, Dorothy's cortisol was likely out of order, based on her stressful job, lack of restorative sleep, and her cravings for carb snacks.

Dorothy's first step was planning regular meals and removing the foods she defaulted from her environment that would ultimately sabotage her. If they're there, you're planning to eat them. She was asked to go to the store with a list, instead of simply buying what looked "good" on the shelves. She began eating foods that increased her level of daytime energy and the amount of her nighttime sleep. Namely, she added lean protein to each meal and eliminated the processed carbs that she was used to consuming. She got used to pairing a fruit with a protein at work to reduce spikes in her level of blood sugar.

Dorothy's downfall was chasing her emotions with food. Socially, she ate. Celebrating, she ate. Stressed, she ate. Typically, her choices were not healthy. A treat never really ended up being a treat, when it was followed with low energy and guilt.

Dealing with her emotions and confronting what was really behind her food choices had to be part of her changing habits. She wasn't used to speaking up for herself. She needed to create a plan and then work the plan. She was very flexible around other people's needs. She had to put herself first. Dorothy was sure that her exercise was the reason she wasn't losing weight, but learned to look at her dietary choices closer for clues. She thought if she skipped a meal and ate snack foods, she'd be better off with fewer calories. Yet, in reality, if she opts to eat less food, it's even more important that she chooses the most nutrient-dense food.

Changing her food habits improved Dorothy's quality and quantity of sleep. It wasn't perfect, but it was better enough that Dorothy did early morning exercise for 20 minutes to build confidence in her ability to be consistent and stick with it. While it wasn't a lot, it was a lot more than nothing. As a result, she had more energy and made better food choices the rest of the day. When she was ready for a more vigorous exercise program, Dorothy got a personal trainer to hold her accountable for showing up and give her the guidance she needed in an intimidating (for her) environment. She is on her way to more muscle and more strength—inside and out.

AFTER 50 FITNESS STRATEGIES: JOANN

In her 60s, JoAnn is not your typical 60-something who decides it's time to exercise. She isn't the type to do too little or to need being motivated. She put in hours of exercise, walking, running, and weightlifting. She would eat as few as 800 calories a day. She didn't take days off. Every day was a "hard" day. Her belief was that the harder and more often she exercised and the less she ate, the more weight she would lose, and the faster she would lose it.

While she didn't lose weight, she did get injured. Two significant injuries within two years finally got her attention. She was breaking her body down, instead of building a stronger, leaner one. She was uniquely classified both as an "athlete," based on her activity level and as obese, based on body composition. Potentially, because of years of ignoring it, she no longer experienced hunger or fullness with any normal pattern. Her physician eliminated the possibility of medical reasons, including thyroid problems.

After strong encouragement, JoAnn began a more varied exercise plan, with hard and easy exercise days. She eventually allowed herself a day off a week. She even boosted her rest periods to two days off a week. It was entirely against everything that she'd ever thought about losing weight.

Gradually, she started to increase her dietary intake to over twice what she once ate. Unlearning old habits and thoughts, such as *fat makes you fat* and *snacking is bad*, she adopted a diet more supportive for an active adult.

Still, with five days a week of what most adults would think of as vigorous exercise and daily healthy eating, JoAnn's weight wouldn't budge. Injury-free and doing everything within her control, her body was still holding onto weight. More medical testing confirmed that her cortisol levels were acceptable.

JoAnn's sleep, however, was both short and disrupted, and had been for over three decades. Waking multiple times a night and sleeping for as little as five hours, she just willed herself to do what she thought had to be done. She was rising at 3 a.m. to fit in exercise at a gym before going to work, which required a drive 45 minutes each way.

With encouragement, she found a gym closer to home, eliminated the 90-minute commute, and shortened her morning exercise period, so that at least she was not rising earlier than 4 a.m. and agreed to be in bed by 9 p.m.

to get seven hours of sleep. That change required time to gradually move bedtime earlier. Still working, JoAnn has a morning deadline and prefers to exercise in the morning.

Under her physician's guidance, JoAnn began a prescription to increase the quality and quantity of her sleep. After trying other possible solutions, this approach was the last resort. She's recording her progress and adjusting the dosage. To date, she's experiencing more quality and quantity sleep than she's had for decades. She's got more energy and focus than she knew possible. Her hunger and satiety cues have returned, even if not as consistently as she'd like. She's now steadily losing weight from a baseline she couldn't budge for a long period of time.

Thirty years of compromised sleep negatively affecting metabolic hormones and years of calorie restriction will take more than a few months to reverse. Still, JoAnn is making progress that has improved her health and quality of life. Continuing on this path she'll add to her 36-pound weight loss.

IF-THEN STRATEGIES WHEN YOU'RE NOT SEEING RESULTS

If your life stressors are up, your exercise intensity, duration, and potentially frequency should go down. Look at both your overall exercise volume and your volume of high-intensity exercise. Remember that too much of any type of exercise (low- or high-intensity) is a cortisol-increasing train on your track.

If you're sleep volume is below your needs, you should reduce the level of your exercise intensity and the duration of your workout. Increase your safety by reducing any demands for agility, reaction skills, and coordination in your exercise routine on the days following poor sleep. Stay ahead of food cravings that are more prevalent after post-sleep deprivation by planning high protein and fiber meals and snacks.

If you're in chronic pain, you should increase the amount of inflammation-reducing foods in your diet and decrease the toxic foods you consume, beginning with sugar. Get more rest and employ more recovery methods than usual. Tell yourself that resting now is your workout.

If you're randomly exercising, you should start planning your high- and low-intensity days with rest days, so that they complement each other. Your exercise needs a purpose, so that your intentions match the outcomes that you want and that your hormones need right now.

If you fear fat, you need to acknowledge it. Start working with your thoughts initially and then your actions. Increasing your intake of healthy fat will reduce your level of inflammation and may reduce your level of bloating (often mistaken for body fat) to help you lose weight. Success breeds confidence. With small changes and adaptations, you'll be able to tackle the next step and the next. You can teach what may now be a carb-and-sugar-burning body how to use fat for fuel. How long have you been eating a higher percent of carbs than protein and fat? It will take a little time, but you can get there.

If you're exercising every day, you should take one full day off once a week. If you take one, but still feel fatigued, add a second day off. You can take them consecutively or separately. Leave at least 48 hours between intense workouts and 72 between heavy weight-training workouts.

If you're choosing foods based on calorie count, you should shift your attention to nutrients. Ignore calories for a period of time. You can always take a snapshot of calories and see how you're doing. If what you're doing is not working, doing more of it is going to dig you a deeper hole.

Are you saying, "I can't _____?" Stop. *I can't lose weight even at 1200 calories a day.* You can't lose weight, because 1200 calories a day is too little for most normal, functioning adult females carrying the weight of the world. *I can't run.* Who said you had to run? *I can't eat breakfast first thing.* Then, don't. Eat as soon as you can. But, consider that you "can't" because you simply haven't before, and it will take some getting used to, but you can. *I can't sleep; I've always had insomnia.* As a baby you slept 14 to 16 hours a day, just like any other baby. You can *improve*.

FEATURED EXPERT: YOU

Now, it's your turn. You're the featured expert on the rest of this story. Only you know your signs and symptoms that something isn't quite right. Only you can take the necessary actions or rest. You got this far. Leap into the appendices, if you haven't yet and begin rewriting your second 50.

APPENDIX A
WORKSHEETS AND FORMS

APPENDIX A-1. THE AFTER 50 PANTRY RAID

Set aside at least an hour to do this exercise so you're not rushed. Then, decide what you're willing to do with the items you don't deem healthy choices for your *After 50 Fitness Formula*. The women's shelter or the food pantry doesn't really need it any more than you do. Can you throw it away? Use one bag or box for throw-away stuff and one for semi-permanent out-of-sight items, while you go through the elimination diet. In that case, remove or hide your wheat and gluten products, sugar, dairy, meat, and higher glycemic load fruits and juices (all but berries and citrus fruit).

- Toss anything with a past expiration date.
- Read your way through every label. Timing consuming, yes. Better that, however, than you consuming foods that are making you fat, sick, or miserable.
- Put all the gluten (refer to the next section), dairy, meat, and sugar items that you have on your shelves in a specific spot. Sugar is better removed completely.
- Read the labels for "extra" items that don't need to be there (i.e., that you shouldn't eat). If you're looking at a peanut butter label, for example, if there's anything but peanut butter (or possibly salt) in it, it really doesn't belong in your body. Tuna should have tuna and water or tuna and oil listed in the ingredients. That's it. Real food is pronounceable and simple.
- Remove anything with trans-fat.
- Check your oils. Move the avocado, olive, coconut, and macadamia nut oils to the front. Throw away the rest.
- Raid your spice rack. Keep what's fresh and toss the rest. Make a list of anything you need, including sea salt, pepper, garlic, cinnamon, turmeric, and garlic powder, as well as ginger, cumin, and oregano, which have gut-healing properties.
- Open the refrigerator and go through the same steps. If anything on the elimination diet can go in the freezer until you know if it's gone permanently or just bye-bye for now, do that. If it's a sugar-filled treat or a fruit-flavored yogurt, toss it. That's never going to be your friend. Don't leave ice cream or Girl Scout Cookies in the freezer. Make it easy to do the right thing and hard to mess it up.
- Finally, open your drawers and cupboards. Are you organized? Do you have go-to items that you can't really get to easily? Move your lesser-used items out of your way. Get your best pans and pots, your high-powered blender, and your grill ready and easy to access. If you could love your kitchen, what would that look like? Do it now. You need to love being in here.
- Done? Take a picture and post to http://www.facebook.com/navigatingfitnessafter50 to share your pantry raid!
- Now, use the Five-Star Foods List (Appendix A-2) to restock. Start with recipes, build your ingredients lists, and go to the store, armed to get everything you need and nothing you don't.

❑ What Is Gluten?

Wheat	Oat	Millet
Rye	Corn	Rice
Barley	Durum	Spelt

❑ Foods Made With Gluten Ingredients

Hot dogs	Canned soups
Luncheon meats	Dried soup mixes
Pickles	Processed cheese
Salad dressings	Cream sauces

Don't be tempted to buy "gluten-free" products without reading the labels. They may not include the highest-quality ingredients. The gluten-free label is just a magnet that marketers hope will attract some buyers. Whole-food options are always a better bet.

❑ Avoid the Following Words on Labels That Allow Producers to Leave Out the Actual Ingredients

Seasoning	Hydrolyzed vegetable protein
Flavoring	Modified food starch
Natural or artificial flavoring	

❑ Sugar by Any Other Name Is Still Sugar

Agave nectar or syrup	Corn sweetener or corn syrup
Barley malt	Date sugar
Beet sugar	Demerara sugar
Blackstrap molasses	Dextran
Brown rice syrup	Diastase
Brown sugar	Ethyl maltol
Buttered sugar	Evaporated cane sugar
Cane juice or cane juice crystals	Fructose
Cane sugar	Fruit juice concentrate
Caramel	Galactose
Carob syrup	Glucose
Castor sugar	Golden sugar
Coconut sugar	Golden syrup

High-fructose corn syrup

Honey

Invert sugar

Lactose

Malt powder

Maltodextrin

Maple syrup

Maltose

Molasses syrup

Muscovado sugar

Oat sugar

Organic raw sugar

Panela

Panocha

Powdered sugar (confectioner's sugar)

Rice bran syrup

Rice syrup

Sorghum and sorghum syrup

Sucrose

Sugar

Syrup

Treacle

Tapioca syrup

Turbinado sugar

Yellow sugar

❏ Artificial Sweeteners

The following list includes the actual name of the artificial sweetener and the obscure names that food companies may be using to hide these ingredients from consumers:

• *Acesulfame Potassium:*

ACK

Ace K

Equal Spoonful (also +aspartame)

Sweet One

Sunett

• *Aspartame:*

APM

AminoSweet (not in the U.S.)

Aspartyl-phenylalanine-1-methyl ester

Canderel (not in the U.S.)

Equal Classic

NatraTaste Blue

NutraSweet

• *Aspartame-Acesulfame Salt:*

TwinSweet (Europe only)

• *Cyclamate (not in the U.S. as per the FDA):*

Calcium cyclamate

Cologran (cyclamate and saccharin) (not in the U.S.)

Sucaryl

- *Erythritol:*

  Sugar alcohol

  Zerose

  ZSweet

- *Glycerol:*

  Glycerin

  Glycerine

- *Glycyrrhizin:*

  Licorice

- *Hydrogenated Starch Hydrolysate (HSH):*

  Sugar alcohol

- *Isomalt:*

  Sugar alcohol

  ClearCut Isomalt

  Decomalt

  DiabetiSweet (also contains Acesulfame-K)

  Hydrogenated Isomaltulose

  Isomaltitol

- *Lactitol:*

  Sugar alcohol

- *Maltitol:*

  Sugar alcohol

  Maltitol Syrup

  Maltitol Powder

  Hydrogenated High Maltose-Content Glucose Syrup

  Hydrogenated Maltose

  Lesys

  MaltiSweet

  SweetPearl

- *Mannitol :*
  Sugar alcohol

- *Neotame Polydextrose:*
  Sugar alcohol (derived from glucose and sorbitol)

- *Saccharin:*

Acid saccharin	Sodium Saccharin
Equal Saccharin	Sweet N Low
Necta Sweet	Sweet Twin

- *Sorbitol:*

  Sugar alcohol
  D-glucitol
  D-glucitol syrup

- *Sucralose:*

1',4,6'-Trichlorogalactosucrose	NatraTaste Gold
Trichlorosucrose	Splenda
Equal Sucralose	

- *Tagatose:*

  Natrulose

- *Xylitol:*

Sugar alcohol	Xylipure
Smart Sweet	Xylosweet

APPENDIX A-2. FIVE-STAR FOODS LIST

This list of nutrient-dense all-stars is designed to get you started. Pick from the list, based on your own food sensitivities and preferences. If you are going through the elimination diet, for instance, you'll leave out dairy, meat, and go light on fruits, even if you usually include them. Suggested menus for eating meatless, dairy-free, or sugar-free can be found at http://foreverfitandfab.com.

❏ Fruits

Apricots	Kiwi
Blackberries	Mango
Blueberries	Peaches
Cantaloupe	Raspberries
Cherries	Strawberries
Citrus fruits (lemon)	

❏ Non-Starchy Vegetables

Artichokes	Kale
Asparagus	Leeks
Avocado (officially a fruit)	Mushrooms
Beets	Onion
Broccoli	Pumpkin
Brussel sprouts	Red pepper
Carrots	Spinach
Cauliflower	Squash
Celery	Sugar snap peas
Cucumber	Tomato
Eggplant	Zucchini
Green beans	

❏ Fiber and Toxin Elimination

Broccoli sprouts
Ground flax seed
Rice bran

❏ Sweetener

    Stevia

❏ High-Quality Protein

    Egg whites and whole eggs   Seafood and fish (low mercury options)
    Lean beef, bison   Skinless white meat
    Low-fat/fat-free cottage cheese   Whey protein isolate
    Low-fat/fat-free Greek yogurt

❏ Plant-Based Protein Sources

    Cannellini and other beans   Quinoa
    Plant-based protein blend   Soy protein isolate

❏ Healthy Fats

    Avocado oil   Extra virgin olive oil
    Chia seed   Nuts and seeds
    Coconut oil

❏ Absorption-Boosting Pre/Probiotics

    Cultured foods
    Fermented foods

❏ Slow-Absorbing Carbs

    Quinoa, brown rice   Sweet potato
    Sprouted wheat tortillas   White kidney beans
    Steel cut oats

❏ Hydration and Liquids

    Chicken or vegetable broth
    Filtered water, green tea
    Milk (dairy, soy, almond, rice, etc.)

APPENDIX A-3. ELIMINATION DIET JOURNAL

The elimination diet is not a calorie-slashing, food-group bashing, hunger-inducing event. There will be temporary elimination of some foods, only to allow some gut healing, as well as create a clean slate. Then, one-by-one, you'll reintroduce foods into your diet and track how you feel.

Remove all of the following triggers for at least a week:

Caffeine*	Soy
Dairy	Sugar
Meat	Wheat/gluten

If you can, continue to follow the elimination diet for three weeks. Sugar is the exception. It's not going to make a comeback. Since alcohol is metabolized as sugar, it's also out. If you want to lose weight, alcohol is not your friend. A minimum of low-glycemic load fruits (e.g., berries and citrus) is acceptable during elimination. You are going to eliminate red meat and poultry. Low mercury fish is encouraged so you can get adequate protein throughout at each meal.

Revisit the pantry raid (Appendix A-1) to get a reminder of where the trigger foods exist, so you can get them both out of sight and out of mind ... as well as out of your mouth. Use the following form to detail any information you subsequently note during elimination:

Start day:

End of week #1:

End of week #2:

End of week #3:

Make comments about any changes in your level of energy, digestion, sleep, or mood that occur during the process.

*You can consume caffeinated coffee as long as you're done drinking it by 10 a.m. If you're extremely stressed and sleep is still evasive once you've completed the rest of the elimination diet, you should consider cutting caffeine out of your diet for a period of time.

By default, you may find that you start eating more green leafy and non-starchy vegetables. That's never a bad thing. Include plenty of healthy fats to your diet by cooking with them, adding them to smoothies, and snacking on nuts and seeds. You should be full, satisfied, and potentially glowing by the end of your elimination diet.

For more information and support concerning how to eliminate toxins from your diet, get *Double Your Energy in 14 Days* at http://foreverfitandfab.com.

❑ Reintroduce One Food at a Time

Eat the food that you're reintroducing to your diet two to three times a day when you bring it back, so you can see that the impact that it has on you right away. Stick with just the one additional food change for three days. Record any reactions you have. If you react poorly, you can stop eating it right away and make a note of how you reacted to this food. At that point, it's something you should avoid. Use the following form to make notes of how you react when you reintroduce a particular food to your diet:

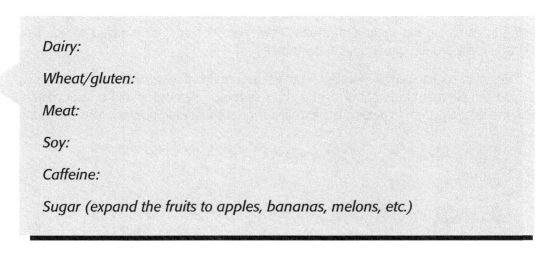

Dairy:

Wheat/gluten:

Meat:

Soy:

Caffeine:

Sugar (expand the fruits to apples, bananas, melons, etc.)

Keep those trigger foods out of your diet for now. In a few months, you may want to try reintroducing them again. You may also find you slip over time, and some of these triggers find their way back into your diet. If it becomes too much for your system, you can go through the elimination diet again with a specific trigger food. Just taking a break from it may be enough for you to heal so you can bring it back into your diet.

APPENDIX A-4. NUTRITION, ACTIVITY, AND PILLOW (NAP) TIME TRACKING

Time of Day & Activity	Details	Comments
5:00 Woke up	Drank big glass of lemon water	
5:15-6:15 Coffee	Writing, answering emails	
6:30 Short run with dog	Light intensity	
7:00 Breakfast	Oatmeal with protein powder, blueberries, walnuts	Hungry, hit the spot
Noon Lunch	Spinach salad, leftover grilled chicken, feta, olives, red wine vinegar	Starving
All afternoon Water	Forgot all morning	Really thirsty all afternoon
4:00 Birthday for someone at work	Wine and cake	Rich! Left work right after
7:00 Dinner	Pasta dinner at friend's home, bread, olive oil	Feeling bloated, heavy, and tired by the time we left
9:00 Bedtime	A little reading	Lights out fast but woke up after a couple hours

Figure A-4a. NAP time tracking blueprint

Use the blueprint in Figure A-4a to keep a record of the time that you arise in the morning, eat, and drink, your level of physical activity, and bedtime. Handwrite it or keep it on your computer. Use something you carry with you to retain this information. Include the content and quantity of the food you eat and details about length and intensity of exercise. Record the three days that represent a normal week for you.

Do this initially before you fill in the 30-day tracker blueprint. The timing and type of food you eat, along with the amount of your sleep and your level of physical activity, can have a big impact on how successful you are in your efforts to enhance your level of energy and lose weight. That's one of the downfalls of online trackers. All they look at is quantity of nutrients and calories according to RDAs, which is a formula that just doesn't serve your needs.

Once you write down your habits, you may see a pattern that isn't serving you well. You can use the following questions to help you in that regard:

- Are you getting 25 to 30 grams of protein at breakfast, lunch, and dinner?
- Are you getting plenty of green leafy and non-starchy vegetables?
- Are you getting snacks that include protein and/or fat to avoid blood sugar spikes?
- Is there healthy fat present in each meal?
- Do you have plenty of time between meals and snacks to digest your food?
- Are you taking in plenty of water regularly between meals?
- Are the carbohydrates you're eating primarily slow-releasing carbs?
- Do you minimize your consumption of processed and packaged foods?

If you're not sure how to interpret your NAP, connect with a health/fitness professional who can provide you with assistance. Get a consultation set up by connecting at http://foreverfitandfab.com.

APPENDIX A-5. SLEEP NEEDS WORKSHEET

Date	Bedtime	Rise Time	Total Hours	Wake Times	Comments

Figure A-5a. Sleep needs chart

The model detailed in Figure A-5a can be used to determine the quality and quantity of your sleep that will enhance your after 50 fitness. The following steps should be utilized to evaluate your sleep needs:

1. Set three to five days aside when you can manipulate the times you go to bed and get up.

2. Record the time you turned out the lights.

3. Include the time you wake naturally.

4. If you remember any wake times or they are reflected on a fitness tracker, even if you don't remember them, make a note of them.

5. Record your total time asleep.

6. In the comments section, record any details. Did you fall asleep easily and feel rested when you woke? How was your energy during the day?

Once you've completed your preliminary sleep needs assessment, you should then do the following:

• Write your usual number of hours of sleep (before the sleep-needs test): _____

• Write your sleep-need number, based on the average of your experiment: _____

• Record any gap between the hours you typically sleep and the number of hours of your ideal sleep: _____

❑ Create a Better Sleep Schedule

Your consistent wake-up time is: _____ (stays the same seven days a week)

Your ideal sleep number is: _____ making your bedtime:_____

Your usual bedtime now: _____

Start by moving bedtime earlier by 20 to 30 minutes per week to adapt. Based on that time, your bedtime for the first week is: _____

Adhere to your efforts to enhance your sleep schedule for a second week and then continue for as many weeks as you need to in order to close your sleep gap.

❑ Create a Bedtime Routine

Refer to the chapter on sleep (Chapter 5) for suggestions beyond eliminating screen time. If bathing or certain relaxing rituals are a part of your current routine or if you have things you want to try, add them to the following list. These cues will begin to tell your body and mind that it's now time to sleep.

- Turn off all screens at (at least 90 minutes before bedtime): _____
-
-
-
-

APPENDIX A-6. 30-DAY AFTER 50 FITNESS TRACKER

Date	RHR	Temp	Water	Sleep	Protein	Fiber	Stress

Figure A-6a. 30-day after 50 fitness tracker

Track your daily numbers on the worksheet for a month, using Figure A-6a. While you're tracking your results, you'll increase your awareness of the importance of these factors. You'll also reinforce good habits, like reaching your goals for optimal levels of fiber, protein, and stress-reducing activities. After 30 days, you'll have enough readings to see a pattern.

You should record a description of the following components:

- *RHR:* Take your resting heart rate the first thing in the morning. If you get up to use the restroom, lie back down, and relax again fully, before taking your heart rate for 15 or 30 seconds. Multiple by four or two, accordingly, to get the number that your heart beats per minute. Alternatively, if you have a heart-rate monitor, you can let it do the work. Take your heart rate before you drink caffeine and as soon after you wake as you can. Changes of 5 to 10 beats a day are significant (refer to Chapter 7 for more information on this topic).

- *Temperature:* Also take your temperature daily the first thing in the morning. Fluctuations above or below normal range can help you track changes, which are potential indications of a thyroid problem that you should share with your physician.

- *Water:* Record the number of eight-ounce glasses of water that you drink daily. Though tea and other fluids count toward hydration, track only the amount of pure water that you drink. It's your best source of hydration.

- *Sleep:* Record your ideal sleep need number (Appendix A-5): _____. On the chart, record your success at meeting this number (e.g., -1, -, +1, etc.). Complete the sleep needs worksheet in Appendix A-5, if you've not already done so.

- *Protein:* Record the number of meals (and/or snacks) you consume that have 25 to 30 grams of protein per day.

- *Fiber:* Record your total grams of daily fiber. In that regard, your minimum goal should be to consume 25 grams. (Between 35 to 50 grams of fiber daily if you have 20 pounds or more to lose.) Increase your existing level by no more than five grams each week to allow your body to slowly adjust to the additional fiber.

- *Stress:* Record the time, in minutes, you dedicate to relaxation and activities that are stress-reducing (not including moderate-to-vigorous exercise time) for you. Sorry—this number should not include screen time!

APPENDIX A-7. THE *AFTER 50 FITNESS FORMULA* INTERVAL WORKSHEET

Your interval options for exercising are infinite, a situation that can be stifling. Keep it simple to begin with. Walk comfortably and walk fast. Bicycle in an easy gear and then increase your level of resistance. There are additional ideas detailed later in this appendix. Then, get as creative as you want. Insert types of exercise, based on your preference. Set up some options that are ready to go, so you don't have to think when you have the time to exercise.

Initially, your longer steady exercise should be in zone 2 (i.e., feels like an RPE of 4 to 5 on a scale of 10) and your 30 seconds should reach zone 4 (i.e., feels like an RPE of 9 on a scale of 10) by the end of the interval. This interval is appropriate for any level of fitness and is an especially good one to start with if you're new to doing intervals.

Interval examples:
- Walk or run the longer interval and then use incline or hill for the 30-second burst.
- Swim or water walk easy and then go as fast as you can.
- Dance in your living room and then do squats or high knee lifts.

Use the following form to detail your 4:30 (easy to moderate) and :30 (hard) interval workout options:

Time:	Activity:
4:30	
:30	
4:30	
:30	
4:30	
:30	
4:30	
:30	

Always perform a warm-up and a cool-down of lighter cardio activity. Include four to eight of the five-minute cycles, both depending on your time constraints and fitness level. Try starting with four intervals and subsequently add one interval a week to the day on which you engage in interval training.

Either to progress or to add variety to your fitness program, shorten the duration of the easy-to-moderate work, while keeping the hard intervals the same duration:

2:00

:30

The rule of thumb is to change one variable at a time. Accordingly, a next progression could be:

2:00

1:00

Once you've adapted to the intervals in your routine, you could do your (easy/hard) 4:30/:30 intervals on Mondays and your 2:00/1:00 on Fridays.

List a few of your own options for easy and hard intervals. Consider your joints, your enjoyment, your goals, and your needs as you are deciding which options to undertake. Among the options that could get you started are the following:

Easy	Hard
Walking	Fast or hill walking
Running	Sprinting or hill running
Swimming	Fast swimming (or harder effort)
Elliptical	Elliptical speed or resistance
Treadmill walking/running	Squats, lunges, chest press, push-ups, etc.
Boxing drills	Faster boxing drills or calisthenics
Hula hoop	Jump rope

Keep in mind that intervals that elevate heart rate do not have to be high-impact and hard on joints. Choose from your many exercise options for safety and results.

APPENDIX A-8. YOUR *AFTER 50 FITNESS FORMULA* RECORDS

The best record of your results is not the scale. Make notes about your levels of energy, sleep, and mood. Find a way to get your body composition measured. If your scale at home doesn't tell you your body fat percentage, a local gym or university may be able to provide you with this measurement. As a rule, this measurement is a simple, non-invasive test, performed either by skinfolds (best done pre- and post-exercise by the same tester) or by bioelectrical impedance. Find out if that's possible, and whether you can return in eight weeks to repeat test.

Weight: _____

Body fat percent: _____

Measurements:

Upper arm: _____ (midway between the elbow and the right shoulder)

Chest: _____ (taken under the bra line)

Belly button: _____ (parallel to the floor, even with the belly button)

Hip: _____ (widest part of the hip, parallel to the floor)

Thigh: _____ (midway between the knee and the right-leg hip)

Calf: _____ (largest part of the calf)

If you feel that you must weigh yourself more than at the start of your exercise routine and subsequently in eight-week intervals, weigh yourself once a week at the same day and time. In addition to the aforementioned measurements, take a picture of yourself, or ask someone to do it for you, in a swimsuit or underwear from the front, back, and side. If you have a full-length mirror, you can take these images easily with a cell phone.

APPENDIX A-9. THE FIVE-DAY PH TRACKER

If you're not feeling right or you lack energy, it can be a lot of things. One of them is that your pH level is too acidic. The pH scale ranges from 0 to 14, 7 being neutral. By testing saliva, you can determine your blood pH level fairly accurately. Your saliva will ideally be 6.5 to 7.0. Use Figure A-9a to track your pH level for five days. Then adjust your diet by increasing the amount of alkaline foods and decreasing the level of acid-producing foods that you consume.

0	1	2	3	4	5	6	7	8	9	10	11	12	13	14

Figure A-9a. The five-day pH tracker

Litmus strips can be obtained either at your local pharmacy or at the following site: https://www.microessentiallab.com/Category/133_1/pH.20_Test.20_Kits.aspx

APPENDIX A-10. WORRY-FREE GRATITUDE JOURNAL

You don't need this book or the research on which it is based to tell you that you have trouble shutting your brain off. You multitask, you tend to worry, and you think about details like you're a boss. All of those qualities make you the amazing person by day that only a woman can be. They can also make it impossible for you to either fall asleep or stay asleep.

Journaling has been proven to be a powerful tool to get your worries on paper and out of your head. Two of the best times to journal are right before bed and right when you rise.

The ritual of journaling is the important factor. You may have nights when it is, in fact, more of a worry journal. You need to write down things so that you don't wake up staring at the ceiling thinking about them in the middle of your stay-young-hormone-releasing time. The other nights, you can focus on a gratitude journal. Either start or end your day by writing 10 things for which you're thankful. At the end of the day, write three things that happened specifically that day for which you have gratitude.

There are no rules for this journal. It's yours. Accordingly, you should feel free to make it up as you go along. When there are big worries or stressors in your life, however, write them down with purpose, as well as an underlying attitude that, *now this is on paper, I can put it to rest until morning.*

Pick up a blank book or grab a simple yellow legal pad. Whichever you do, dedicate it just to journaling and leave it at your bedside. If you're not a natural at maintaining a journal, give yourself a prompt to start your efforts to record your day-to-day inner thoughts.

What 10 things am I grateful for today?

1.

2.

3.

4.

5.

6.

7.

8.

9.

10.

Three things that happened today for which I'm thankful:

1.

2.

3.

Things I want to remember for tomorrow:

1.

2.

3.

APPENDIX A-11. STRESS TOOLBOX WORKSHEET

Stress is personal, specific, and individual. For each kind of stressful experience you encounter, you may need a different tool to fix it. For example, you don't need stitches for a mosquito bite. You might need an ice pack for a swollen ankle.

Take time to identify your biggest stressors. Then, choose from the list of ideas and expand to your own list of stress Rx. The underlying concept is to reduce stress by including stress-reduction activities before you're bleeding.

What are your biggest sources of stress? (Be specific.)

1.

2.

3.

4.

5.

Write down one thing for each of those stressors that would help reduce or eliminate it:

1.

2.

3.

4.

5.

Circle any of the items on this list that appeal to you. Add your own set of hobbies, rituals, or activities to it.

- Listening to music (Try www.wholetones.com)
- Meditation
- Nature walking
- Photography
- Painting, drawing, or other artistic hobby
- Exercise, dancing, or leisure-time sport
- Time with friends
- Time with a pet
- Getting away regularly (mini-vacation)

- Private time with a partner or spouse
-
-
-

Consider realistically when you can add some of your stress reducers to your regular schedule. Lastly, but most importantly, what has to go, so that you have time to dedicate to taking care of yourself?

1.

2.

3.

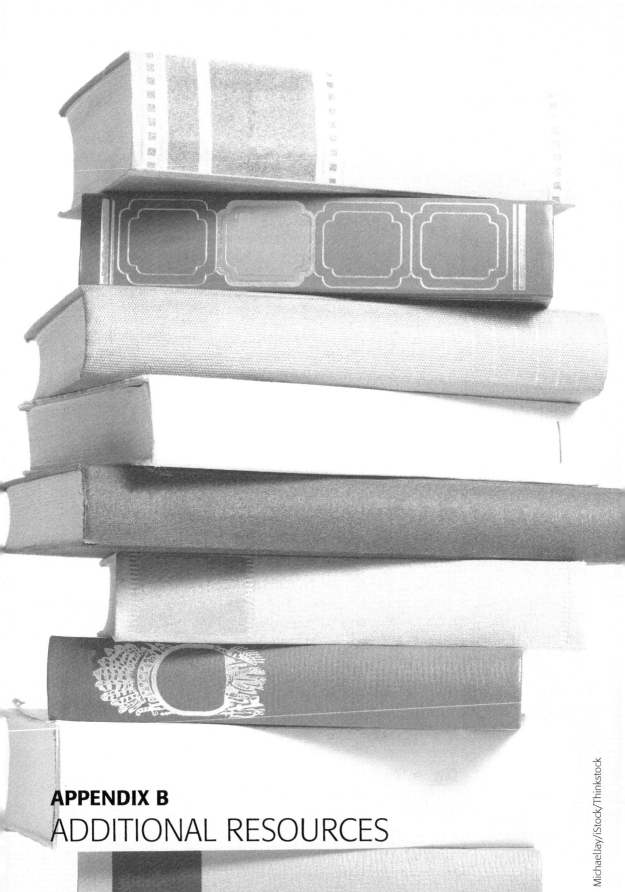

APPENDIX B
ADDITIONAL RESOURCES

APPENDIX B-1. PROTEIN POWDER PRIMER

Getting enough high-quality protein, as well as getting it while your muscles are most in need of it, is important to an after 50 woman who wants to keep the best bod and a life as active as possible.

Getting the majority of your protein needs met from whole foods, ideally from a mixture of animal and plant sources, would require you to eat a lot of chicken and salmon, or huge amounts of beans, rice, and quinoa to include plant-only proteins. Fortunately, protein supplements are convenient and economical, as well as good-tasting in many instances. You do, however, have to watch for sugars and artificial sweeteners. Limit yourself to consuming two to three grams of sugar per serving, if possible, and if there's an artificial sweetener used, select stevia, if possible.

There are a lot of terms to consider on the protein supplement shelves these days. Product labels can be confusing. There is a difference in the quality of the products that makes it worth your research. You need to know a couple key terms to get you started in the right direction. If you're choosing protein from plant-based products, there are also a couple key ingredients to making an optimal choice, which are usually listed toward the bottom of the label.

❑ Dairy Proteins

- *Whey or casein concentrate:* This substance is the cheapest form of protein supplement. Because it's only about 80 percent protein, it has more fat and carbs as "fillers." It is harder to mix and doesn't dissolve as well as higher-quality options, but it still offers muscle-building benefits.
- *Isolate:* This is more processed, i.e., which removes the fats and carbs, has 90 to 95 percent protein, and dissolves much better.
- *Hydrosylate or hydrolyzed protein:* This option has been broken down into smaller, more easily absorbed parts and gets into the muscles faster.
- *Micellar casein or isolated casein:* This expensive option is easy to mix and is almost pure casein—the slower-acting protein that is most beneficial when it is ingested at bedtime or taken as a meal replacement (note: it is not recommended if whole-food protein is readily available).
- *Milk protein:* 80 percent casein and 20 percent whey.
- *Egg white protein:* An excellent high-quality protein, often higher in price compared to others. The term "instantized egg albumin" may be how it is listed on the label.
- *"Proprietary blend":* Consumers need to be fully aware of the fact that supplement companies don't have to disclose what mixture of whey, casein, and "other" ingredients they use in their products.

❑ Plant Proteins

- *Soy:* This substance is high-quality protein, with all the amino acids needed for muscle growth. If you're worried about including soy, due to its effect on estrogen, be aware of the fact that most of the soy isoflavones causing the interaction with human hormones have been removed from soy isolate.
- *Hemp:* This substance has all of the essential amino acids, but is low in leucine, which is the most important amino acid for protein synthesis. In other words, if you're taking the protein to reach the amounts necessary to maintain your muscle mass, this particular protein source doesn't give you the boost you want. It does provide a significant amount of fiber and healthy fat, however.
- *Brown rice:* This substance is also low in leucine, but it does offer vegans and vegetarians a viable source of protein.
- *Yellow pea:* This substance may be helpful in reducing your appetite, but it is also low in leucine.
- *Plant-based protein blend:* These products mix different plant sources of protein to provide a protein with the appropriate dose of leucine.

It is important to know that plant-based proteins generally have a more grainy or chalky texture, and none to date have a great taste by themselves. As a result, you may want to add it to a smoothie, with fruit or vegetables that can help it become more palatable.

The essential amino acids leucine, isoleucine, and valine (particularly leucine) are more important than the other 17 (20 total) amino acids in assisting protein synthesis, muscle growth, and repair. It takes two to three grams of leucine for maximum protein synthesis. A meal of eggs, fish, meat, or a smoothie made with carefully selected protein powder can do that. Figure B-1a illustrates a comparison of approximately how many grams of each of the selected proteins you need to get 2.5 grams of leucine.

Protein	Grams
Whey	23
Egg	29
Soy	31
Rice	32
Pea	39
Hemp	100

Figure B-1a. Leucine per grams of protein type

It's easy to see why whey protein is the most popular type of protein. It's convenient, as well as gives you exactly what you need in each serving.

At this point, you may have concerns that your whey protein (it is dairy, after all) can make you fat. If you follow the guidelines for selecting the highest quality protein powders, you'll have less chance of experiencing problems. Try a small container before walking out of a store with one that will last months. If you've been using whey and can't lose weight despite checking all of the other factors (sleep, stress, other foods) that it could be, remove whey from your diet for at least one week and perhaps up to three weeks. See what happens and how you feel. Subsequently, reintroduce it to your diet to see how you're affected. If whey is part of the reason that is preventing you from achieving your desired weight loss, you should see some difference from elimination and reintroduction.

APPENDIX B-2. HIGH-QUALITY PROTEIN SOURCES AND SERVING SIZES

Anchovies – 24 g per 3 oz.

Canned crab – 22 g per 6.5 oz. can

Chicken or turkey breast – 35 g per 4 oz.

Ground beef – 28 g per 4 oz.

Ground chicken – 26 g per 4 oz.

Ground turkey – 22 g per 4 oz.

Halibut – 25 g per 4 oz.

Light canned tuna – 22 g per 4 oz.

Salmon – 29 g per 4 oz.

Sardines – 22 g per 3.75 oz. can

Shrimp – 24 g per 4 oz.

Tilapia – 26 g per 4 oz.

Top or bottom beef steak – 34 g per 4 oz.

Tuna (bluefin) steak– 34 g per 4 oz.

❑ Additional Sources of Protein

Cottage cheese – 14 g per ½ cup

Greek Yogurt – 23 g per 8 oz. serving

Hard cheese (cheddar, Swiss, etc.) – 7 g per 1 oz.

Organic cows or soy milk – 8 g per 1 cup serving

Pastured eggs – 6 g per 1 large egg

Protein powders – vary a great deal (read more in Appendix B-1)

❑ Plant-Based Sources of Protein

Mixed nuts – 6 g per 2 oz. serving

Peanut Butter – 8 g per 2 tbsp.

Quinoa – 8 g per 1 cup serving

White kidney beans (most beans) – 15 g per 1 cup

APPENDIX B-3. THE *AFTER 50 FITNESS FORMULA* SMOOTHIE PLAN

Make a delicious and nutritious meal or snack with whole-food and high-quality protein that will boost the level of fiber, healthy fat, and antioxidants in your diet. Come up with your own variations following this simple formula. Keep in mind that because blended foods are already partially broken down, more of the nutrients are easily absorbed.

- Liquid: water, milk (cow's, almond, or soy), hemp, coconut, green tea
- Protein powder: whey, planted-based blend, soy, Greek yogurt, white kidney beans
- Veggies: spinach/kale/chard, pumpkin/sweet potato/squash, beets, cucumber/celery
- Fruit: berries (lowest in sugar), apple, pear, pineapple, banana
- Healthy fat: nuts, nut butter, ground flax/chia/hemp seeds, avocado
- Spice or flavor (optional): cinnamon, nutmeg, coconut, pure vanilla

If you're trying to lose weight or working on the elimination diet, use berries as your fruit to keep the sugar content of your diet low. Don't skimp on the level of healthy fat. Choose your solid ingredients first and then add just enough liquid for the thickness you want.

❏ Sweet Green Smoothie

- 2 celery stalks
- Handful of romaine
- Handful of spinach
- Fresh-squeezed lemon
- Green apple
- Parsley
- Pear
- Ripe banana

Blend the celery, romaine, and spinach. Add the remaining ingredients, cover with water, and add ice. Halve the fruits to reduce the amount of sugar. This smoothie is a good first-thing-in-the-morning drink for reducing acidity and boosting antioxidants.

❏ Can't Beet That Smoothie

- 1 c. water
- ½ medium avocado
- 2 celery stalks
- 1 c. frozen strawberries
- 1 medium beet, cooked or prepared
- 1 lemon, juiced
- 1 tbsp. coconut oil
- 4 ice cubes
- 1 apple, cored
- Protein powder (unflavored or vanilla)

Combine all of the ingredients and blend. Beets are powerful antioxidants that help the body naturally detox and help reduce inflammation. They're naturally sweet, so you may be pleasantly surprised if beets are a new addition to smoothies for you.

❏ Recovery Smoothie

- 1 c. almond or coconut milk
- ½ c. frozen or fresh berries
- ½ frozen banana
- 1 tsp. honey
- Dash of cinnamon
- Small handful of almonds/cashews (or nut butter)
- Scoop of protein powder (chocolate or vanilla)
- Chia seeds
- Ground flax
- Optional: add a handful of spinach or ½ avocado

Blend. Loaded with antioxidants and anti-inflammation ingredients, this high-fiber smoothie will help you recover after your workout.

❏ Pumpkin Pie Smoothie

- 1 c. almond milk
- ½ c. pumpkin puree
- 4 ice cubes
- 4 Medjool dates, pitted
- ¼ tsp. pure vanilla extract
- ¼ tsp. ground cinnamon
- Pinch of pumpkin pie spice
- Scoop of vanilla protein powder

Combine all ingredients and blend. Because the dates increase the sugar content, this smoothie is best immediately post-exercise, when you're replenishing your energy stores. Wonderfully creamy fall treat.

APPENDIX B-4. SAFE FISH

Fish is recommended as a lean protein source and many fish options contain healthy omega 3 fats. You want to keep a watch on toxic mercury levels in the fish choices you make. In general, wild caught, local options are best. Use the following link to help you make informed decisions on fish: http://www.nrdc.org/health/effects/mercury/walletcard.pdf

APPENDIX B-5. RECOVERY RESOURCES

❏ Foam Rollers

http://www.power-systems.com/s-67-foam-rollers.aspx

❏ The Stick

https://www.thestick.com

❏ Heart Rate Variability Monitors

http://www.bioforcehrv.com

APPENDIX B-6. BOOKS FOR ADDITIONAL READING

Age Is Just a Number: Achieve Your Dreams at Any Stage in Your Life—Dara Torres

Body-for-LIFE for Women—Pamela M. Peeke

Fight Fat After Forty—Pamela M. Peeke

Grain Brain—David Perlmutter and Kristin Loberg

The Adrenal Reset Diet—Alan Christianson

The Female Brain—Daniel Amen

The Healthiest Meals on Earth—Jonny Bowden

The Hormone Reset Diet—Sara Gottfried

The Hunger Fix: The Three-Stage Detox and Recovery Plan for Overeating and Food Addiction—Pamela M. Peeke

The Metabolic Effect—Jade Teta

The Sugar Impact Diet—JJ Virgin

Wheat Belly—William Davis

APPENDIX B-7. SUPPLEMENT SOLUTIONS

The following list details a collection of the most recommended natural (versus synthetic) supplements by physicians for women's health. Many of these supplements have been mentioned throughout the book, specifically for their ability to help boost sleep, improve hormone function, or enhance gut health. By no means inclusive, this list is provided as a recommendation. Rather, it is intended to serve as possibly a good point to start a conversation on the topic with your physician. It is also important to be aware of the fact that you should always check with your physician regarding interactions with medications and supplementation recommendations specific to you.

- A multivitamin (one tablet, twice a day)
- Fish oil (2000 mg a day)
- Probiotics (10 to 60 billion CFUs)
- Calcium citrate (400 to 500 mg twice a day)
- Chelated magnesium (250 to 600 mg daily/200 to 300 mg twice a day)
- Vitamin D (2000 IU of D3, taken in addition to a multivitamin)
- Zinc (15 mg)

In addition to natural supplements, it is also important to be aware of the fact that selenium, vitamin D, vitamin A, iron, zinc, copper, and vitamin C are essential to the health of your thyroid. Iodine is also important. Because it can be toxic, however, you should be tested for the level of iodine in your body before supplementation. In addition to the aforementioned, your body may also need the following supplements (check with your physician before taking):

- Melatonin (3 to 6 mg taken at night 90 minutes before bedtime to aid sleep)
- DHEA (if needed, 50 to 100 mg 7-Keto-DHEA)
- N-acetylcysteine (NAC) (600 mg once or twice daily; supports liver detox efforts and brain health)

❑ Spices

Experiment with spices as you cook. Be open to herbs used in ayurvedic medicine (i.e., holistic healing system), but also be aware of their potential interaction with medications you may be taking. When in doubt, check with your physician first.

Cinnamon helps to balance your level of blood sugar. You need to be generous if you're sprinkling this spice on your oatmeal or adding it to a smoothie or soup. You want to use at least ¼ to 1¼ teaspoons.

Another spice, turmeric, can improve your gut health. It can also prevent the additional production of cortisol by deactivating an enzyme that is able to convert inactive cortisone to cortisol. Cooling with turmeric once or twice a week, however, isn't enough to provide these health benefits. You'll also need 80 to 500 milligrams of curcumin, which is the key active ingredient in turmeric, on a daily basis, along with its sidekick black pepper, which boosts curcumin absorption in the bloodstream, to achieve gut health and decrease cortisol production. In fact, you'd need to eat two to four grams of turmeric daily, along with an adequate amount of black pepper, to ingest the desired level of curcumin in turmeric. Continue spice your life with turmeric. A curcumin supplement, however, may be a more reasonable way to get adequate levels of curcumin. On the off chance that cortisol is not a concern for you and that you're focused on gut healing alone, you don't need the black pepper to enhance curcumin absorption in your bloodstream.

Several other spices will enhance your enjoyment of foods, while they also boost your level of metabolism. Experiment with metabolic favorites, like ginger, cayenne, and mustard. Don't stop there, since many spices will make your eating experience more pleasurable and add an array of health benefits, while they do so.

❑ Herbs

Several herbs are often discussed with regard to women's health, without consistency in message, either across the literature or among the experts. The following two herbs, however, stand out as the most frequently recommended by leading authorities on women's health:

- Ashwagandha (250 mg two to three times a day; promotes thyroid health and optimal cortisol levels)
- Chasteberry (20 to 40 mg a day; decreases PMS-like symptoms of irritability, mood disturbances, and headache)

APPENDIX B-8. MUSCLES IN MINUTES: 10-MINUTE SEQUENCES

These sequences can be done in endless combinations. Short on time or just starting out? Complete just one set (i.e., one time through) of a single sequence. Have more time and have a basic foundation of muscular fitness? Complete a sequence two or three times.

Each set of an exercise will take about a minute, no matter how you look at it. If you're doing a light weight, you'll perform about 12 to 15 repetitions of each exercise. If you're doing a heavy weight, you may fatigue at fewer than 10 repetitions. As such, you should incorporate a little rest between exercises. For videos of these and other exercises, visit www.youtube.com/allagesfitness.

For more variety you can mix up the sequences. Perform one set each of sequences #1, #2 and #3 for a 10-minute workout. You can repeat the routine of performing one set of three separate sequences two or three times if you have more time, as well as the fitness foundation to do more.

❑ Sequence #1

- Squats
- Chest press
- Standing bent-over row

❑ Sequence #2

- Lunges (alternating rear lunges)
- One-arm chest press
- Single-arm bent-over row

❑ Sequence #3

- Single-leg dead lift
- Alternating arm chest press
- Bent-arm pullover (in a gym: lat pull down, seated or standing row)

The aforementioned sequences each feature compound exercises that are designed to engage the major muscle groups of the body. Because this type of exercise has the greatest impact on your level of metabolism, they should be your highest priority. When you have more time, you can expand your exercise routine to include the smaller muscle groups that are addressed in sequences #4 and #5. Keep in mind that because the exercises in sequences #1, #2, and #3 also stimulate the smaller muscles of the body, you shouldn't feel that you need to do all of the exercises every day.

❑ Sequence #4

- Bicep curls
- Tricep press
- Bridge

❑ Sequence #5 (hint: use light resistance)

- Front raise
- Lateral raise
- Reverse fly

❑ Make It Cardio

To add a cardio aspect to any of the aforementioned sequences (i.e., #s 1-5), incorporate two minutes of aerobic activity after each set of three exercises. For example, hop on the treadmill, spin, use a hula hoop, or do boxing drills. Anything that elevates your heart rate will work. Then, either repeat the same scenario or undertake a new one. The point is to continue doing three exercises and then two minutes of cardio for whatever time you want to exercise.

APPENDIX B-9. SNACK SUCCESS STRATEGIES

There's no need to snack if you feel at the top of your game with three squares and no snacks. In some cases, not snacking will be best for your hormones. For those times when you need something, a snack of protein + carb + fat is a good formula. A carb alone will spike your blood sugar, even if it's a nutrient-dense fruit, particularly if it's been awhile since you last ate.

❑ If an early start means at least five hours to lunch, mid-morning snack:
  • Chia pudding
  • Greek yogurt and berries
  • Half a piece of fruit (pear/apple) with string cheese
  • Hummus and carrots or cucumbers

❑ Control mid/late afternoon cravings with a high protein snack by 2 p.m.:
  • Almonds (about 20)
  • A small protein shake (low sugar)
  • Celery and almond butter
  • Sunflower seeds
  • Two hard-boiled eggs
  • Walnuts

❑ If it's been hours since lunch, pre-exercise snack*:
  • Half a banana with a little nut butter
  • Milk** or water, with protein powder
  • Small Greek yogurt,** with fresh berries

❑ Post vigorous exercise or strength training snack, if it's more than 90 minutes to a meal:
  • Chocolate milk or soy milk (eight grams of protein per serving)
  • Simple whey protein in either water or milkshake***

❑ If it's been three hours since dinner and you're hungry before bed snack:
  • Small protein shake (casein would be more ideal than whey)
  • Walnuts or almonds

---

*Nutritionists suggest that stomach clearing is the single most important factor in choosing pre-exercise snacks, so that your digestion and muscles aren't fighting for the available blood flow. Pre-exercise is not a good time to add fiber. If you're weight training or doing Pilates, as opposed to jogging, your stomach you may be able to handle a little more fat. Some fitness experts suggest eating peanut butter or avocado before exercise. Experiment with what works for you.
**If you're going to engage in something aerobic or intense exercise, you should leave dairy out of your diet.
***Don't overuse protein drinks, when you have access to real food, as well as time to eat.

Be sure to snack wisely to help you get more vegetables, low sugar fruits, high-quality protein, and healthy fat into your diet. Eating in a fast-paced life, mandates that you make everything count in your diet.

APPENDIX B-10. TESTING YOUR HORMONE HEALTH

When you've assessed your lifestyle from all angles, made changes, and still don't feel right, it's time to test. The following tests may help fill in the blanks for you about what might be negatively affecting your level of metabolism and energy. You can ask your physician about testing or find online labs for testing and order your own, for example, www.mymedlab.com or www.healthtestingcenters.com.

❑ Complete Blood Count and Metabolic Panel (fasting blood test)

- White and red blood count, cholesterol, and glucose

❑ Ferritin (blood test)

- If you're experiencing signs of anemia, e.g., fatigue, breathlessness, etc., ask specifically for this test. Low levels of ferritin are often associated with anemia, while levels that are too high are not ideal either.

❑ Vitamin D (blood test)

- Vitamin D deficiency is related to obesity, depression, cognitive impairment, and reduced immunity.

❑ Iodine (blood test)

- You need iodine for good thyroid function, yet it can also be potentially toxic. Accordingly, if you suspect you're not getting enough iodine in your diet, you should be tested.

❑ Thyroid (blood test)

- Be proactive in your health and ask your physician about how you fare on certain measures of thyroid health, including TSH, thyroid antibodies (TG and TPO), thyroglobin, and reverse T3. If your ranges appear "normal," but your symptoms persist, you may need to undergo an ultrasound.

❑ Cortisol and DHEA-S (blood and saliva test)

- Both control and DHEA-S are adrenal gland stress hormones. Saliva testing is done at four different times of the day to determine how your cortisol levels compare to an optimal level of cortisol.

❑ Estrogen and Progesterone (blood or saliva)

- Ideally, both hormones should be in balance, relative to each other, as well as within their normal ranges. Even post-menopause, you can be estrogen-dominant, resulting in different symptoms and strategies.

❑ Testosterone (blood test)

- Yes, even as a woman, you want optimal testosterone levels to feel and look great.

❑ Food Allergy (blood test)

- You should also be aware of the fact that you may have mild allergies, which means that you can still eat a particular food without unduly reacting. On the other hand, you may be more comfortable or experience a higher level of energy without consuming that food.

Notes

The bibliography for *You Still Got It, Girl! The After 50 Fitness Formula for Women* is available on a page on my website in tree-sparing spirit. Please visit this link to see the research sources: http://foreverfitandfab.com/you-still-got-it-girl-the-book/book-resources

About the Author

Debra Atkinson is the founder of Voice for Fitness, LLC. She first began her career in the fitness industry in 1984, and, since that time, has led thousands of fitness classes, conducted thousands of personal training sessions, managed group-fitness classes, and supervised over 200, 000 personal training sessions as director of programming. She served as a senior lecturer in kinesiology at Iowa State University, where she taught 14 years. She has also been a private wellness coach for over 18 years. She uses the science of fitness, together with the art of exercise psychology, to create programs that work.

Over her 30-year career, Debra has:
- Been a subject matter expert for the American Council on Exercise (ACE)
- Presented for IDEA Health & Fitness Association, Can-Fit-Pro, National Strength & Conditioning Association (NSCA), and the International Council on Active Aging
- Written over 250 articles for various organizations, including IDEA and NSCA
- Served as the captain for the Live Healthy Iowa Dream Team, as well as speaker and challenge administrator for the American Heart Association's Go Red For Women
- Spoken to thousands of audiences about the art and science of finding their "fit"

In addition to her experience in fitness, coaching, writing, and speaking, Debra takes the time to walk the talk. She is a five-time Ironman starter, a four-time finisher in that challenging event, and a barely boomer that can connect with an audience of one or 1000.

She has the dual blessings of calling Iowa home and living in Boulder, Colorado. Her son, Dustin, is a business major and member of the men's golf team at the University of Northern Iowa.

For more information about Debra, you can visit http://foreverfitandfab.com, or reach out to her After 50 community on Facebook and Twitter at:

Facebook: http://www.facebook.com/navigatingfitnessafter50

Twitter: https://www.twitter.com/after50fitness

Send Debra your question or challenge at http://Flipping50TV.com